Refraction and Reti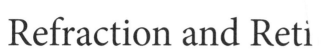

Refraction and retinoscopy are essential skills in progression through ophthalmology specialty training and require consistent practice. This second edition is a comprehensive introduction and revision guide specifically tailored for candidates sitting the Refraction Certificate, as assessed by the Royal College of Ophthalmologists.

Key features:

- Presents concise explanations of the theory and application of refraction and retinoscopy techniques, with excellent guided illustrations throughout.
- Provides a step-by-step framework for how best to prepare for the recently updated format of the Refraction Certificate.

MasterPass Series

Advanced ENT Training: A Guide to Passing the FRCS (ORL-HNS) Examination
Joseph Manjaly, Peter Kullar

The Final FRCR: Self-Assessment
Amanda Rabone, Benedict Thomson, Nicky Dineen, Vincent Helyar, Aidan Shaw

Geriatric Medicine: 300 Specialist Certificate Exam Questions
Shibley Rahman, Henry Woodford

Clinical Cases for the FRCA: Key Topics Mapped to the RCoA Curriculum
Alisha Allana

MCQs, MEQs and OSPEs in Occupational Medicine: A Revision Aid
Ken Addley

ENT Vivas: A Guide to Passing the Intercollegiate FRCS (ORL-HNS) Viva Examination
Adnan Darr, Karan Jolly, Jameel Muzaffar

ENT OSCEs: A Guide to Your First ENT Job and Passing the MRCS (ENT) OSCE
Peter Kullar, Joseph Manjaly, Livy Kenyon

Plastic Surgery Vivas for the FRCS (Plast): An Essential Guide
Monica Fawzy

Neurosurgery Second Edition: The Essential Guide to the Oral and Clinical Neurosurgical Exam
Vivian Elwell, Ramez Kirollos, Syed Al-Haddad, Peter Bodkin

The Final FFICM Structured Oral Examination Study Guide
Eryl Davies

Refraction and Retinoscopy: How to Pass the Refraction Certificate, Second Edition
Jonathan Park, Leo Feinberg, David Jones

For more information about this series, please visit: https://www.routledge.com/MasterPass/book-series/CRCMASPASS

Refraction and Retinoscopy

How to Pass the Refraction Certificate

Second Edition

Jonathan C. Park, Leo J. Feinberg,
and David H. Jones

Illustrations supervised by Salman Waqar

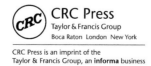

CRC Press
Taylor & Francis Group
Boca Raton London New York

CRC Press is an imprint of the
Taylor & Francis Group, an **informa** business

Designed cover image: Shutterstock

Second edition published 2024
by CRC Press
6000 Broken Sound Parkway NW, Suite 300, Boca Raton, FL 33487-2742

and by CRC Press
4 Park Square, Milton Park, Abingdon, Oxon, OX14 4RN

CRC Press is an imprint of Taylor & Francis Group, LLC

© 2024 Jonathan Park, Leo J. Feinberg, David Jones and Salman Waqar

First edition published by Radcliffe Publishing 2003

Library of Congress Cataloging-in-Publication Data
Names: Park, Jonathan C., author. | Jones, David H. (Ophthalmologist), author. | Feinberg, Leo J., author.
Title: Refraction and retinoscopy : how to pass the refraction certificate / Jonathan C. Park, Leo J. Feinberg, David H. Jones ; illustrations supervised by Salman Waqar. Other titles: Master pass. Description: 2nd edition. | Boca Raton : CRC Press, 2024. | Series: Master pass | Includes bibliographical references and index. | Identifiers: LCCN 2023023090 (print) | LCCN 2023023091 (ebook) | ISBN 9781032359137 (hardback) | ISBN 9781032359120 (paperback) | ISBN 9781003329329 (ebook)
Subjects: MESH: Refraction, Ocular | Refractive Errors | Retinoscopy–methods | Study Guide
Classification: LCC RE925 (print) | LCC RE925 (ebook) | NLM WW 18.2 | DDC 617.7/55–dc23/eng/20230816
LC record available at https://lccn.loc.gov/2023023090
LC ebook record available at https://lccn.loc.gov/2023023091

ISBN: 9781032359137 (hbk)
ISBN: 9781032359120 (pbk)
ISBN: 9781003329329 (ebk)

DOI: 10.1201/9781003329329

Typeset in Minion
by Newgen Publishing UK

Contents

Forewords

Refraction is a difficult but really important skill to embrace. It's a satisfying examination technique that not only enhances your patient assessments and your diagnostic abilities but can also help you problem-solve and reassure patients in eye casualty and clinics. It's so important that the Royal College of Ophthalmologists have for a long time made it an essential skill, with the Refraction Certificate being compulsory for progression within specialist training.

It can seem like a dark art, however, and one that can be difficult to pick up along the way. This book provides a really clear description of the skills that you will need to demonstrate, both for your exam and in clinical practice. It has been updated to include the COVID and post-COVID modifications of the RCOphth exam, and provides a really useful framework on which to base your exam preparation.

Written by your colleagues who are educationalists and ophthalmologists, and who have all had to learn these same skills, this book is an excellent practical guide to direct your practice, simulation, and reading.

Ms Tamsin Sleep FRCOphth
Consultant Ophthalmologist
Head of School, Ophthalmology
NHS South West Peninsula Deanery
June 2023

Refraction is an art that requires time and perseverance to master. This updated textbook continues on from the first edition by describing concisely the most commonly used refraction techniques and has excellent instructions to aid in preparation for the Royal College examinations. The authors describe both objective and subjective methods of refraction with good instructions on how to interpret the results. There is a wealth of clinical pearls. This practical textbook will continue to act as a favourite benchmark for all ophthalmology trainees and practitioners, or anyone keen to learn the 'Art of Refraction'. I congratulate the authors on their efforts.

Mr Indy S Sian FRCOphth, Cert LRS, PGCert (Clin Ed), MCOptom
Consultant Ophthalmic Surgeon
RCOphth Examiner & College Tutor
June 2023

Acknowledgements

The authors thank the Royal College of Ophthalmologists for their permission to publish this text with their material. We are also hugely grateful to Mr Salman Waqar, Consultant Ophthalmic Surgeon, for his illustrations, and Dr David Adams, Senior Optometrist at University Hospitals Plymouth, for his insights and review.

About the authors

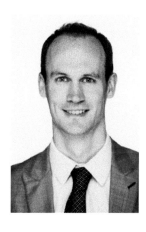

Jon Park has worked in Somerset as a Consultant Ophthalmic Surgeon since 2015. He graduated from the University of Bristol, UK, and then completed his specialty training in the South West Peninsula Deanery. He subsequently completed a vitreo-retinal surgical fellowship at the University of Toronto, Canada.

Jon's main research interests relate to training and various aspects of cataract and vitreo-retinal surgery including post-operative infections. He has presented his research work at over 60 conferences across the UK, Europe, and North America. He has published over 30 research articles in peer-reviewed journals and is the author of three ophthalmic textbooks relating to training. His previous research projects have been awarded the international Global Ophthalmology Awards Program and the Royal College of Ophthalmologists' Fight for Sight Award. Currently, Jon is a member of the Royal College's scientific committee panel, the British Ophthalmological Surveillance Unit (BOSU).

Jon is keen on training and is a Royal College educational and clinical supervisor. He hopes that the second edition of this book will help ophthalmic surgeons develop their practical refraction skills by focusing on the parts of refraction an ophthalmic surgeon needs – for their exams and their clinics.

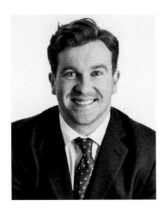

Leo Feinberg is a fourth-year specialty trainee in ophthalmology in the Peninsula Deanery. He graduated from the University of Birmingham with honours in both Medical Sciences and Medicine and Surgery. He undertook the Academic Foundation Programme in Medical Management and Leadership in the West Midlands, during which he completed his Membership of the Royal College of Surgeons before joining the Ophthalmology specialty training program in Peninsula. He has completed his FRCOphth examinations and is now completing a Postgraduate Certificate in Medical Management and Leadership through the University of Keele.

Whilst the first edition of this text was invaluable for his preparation for the Refraction Certificate, he realised that contemporary text was lacking. He hopes this second edition becomes a close companion for any candidate preparing for the refraction exam.

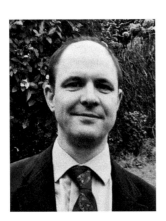

David Jones is a full-time Consultant Ophthalmologist in Cornwall. He studied medicine at Cambridge and Oxford Universities and undertook most of his ophthalmology training in Glasgow. He is an educational supervisor for ophthalmic trainees in Cornwall.

Abbreviations

BD	base-down
BI	base-in
BO	base-out
BU	base-up
BVD	back vertex distance
cyl	cylinder
IPD	inter-pupillary distance
JCC	Jackson cross cylinder
MR	Maddox rod
OSCE	objective structured clinical examination
OST	Ophthalmic Specialty Training
PCT	prism cover test
pd	prism dioptre

1

Introduction – A book for junior doctors and optometrists

Refraction, like most practical skills, is an art with a scientific basis. Once mastered, it is satisfying for the practitioner and patient. However, learning to refract is often bewildering. The authors found that when starting to learn refraction, everybody would tell them that practice was the key. We agree strongly with this, but initially, the obvious question is – 'practice what?' Therefore, learners tend to turn to large textbooks not typically tailored to the junior ophthalmologist or optometrist.

The aim of this handbook is to provide a concise and simple understanding of the refractive process. This will give the reader confidence, and rather than waste time getting confused in large textbooks, allow them to pick their retinoscope up at an earlier stage.

This book has been written for anyone preparing to take the 'Refraction Certificate'. This includes junior ophthalmologists who have already passed the Royal College of Ophthalmologists' Part 1 examination, but also junior doctors and medical students, keen to get ahead in preparation for their Ophthalmic Specialty Training applications, but who have less clinical experience in ophthalmology. It will also serve as a revision aid for those taking the Part 1 examination, who are keen to link theory to practice whilst revising.

We also hope that this book is useful to every junior optometrist and any senior ophthalmologist who has let their refractive skills slip and needs a brief reminder of how to revive this technique.

We hope that this latest edition will bear fruit for candidates undertaking the updated format of the Refraction Certificate examination as of 2022 and any future formats thereafter.

Jonathan C Park, Leo J Feinberg, and David H Jones
June 2023

DOI: 10.1201/9781003329329-1

2

The Refraction Certificate examination

The Refraction Certificate examination has undergone several iterations since it began. The most recent came in 2020 due to the COVID pandemic, whereby all patient-facing stations were replaced by simulated retinoscopy performed on model eyes. Examinations were performed in isolation with no examiners present, and all answers were manually entered onto an iPad answer form. At the time of writing this, the College has updated the Refraction Certificate examination to a hybrid format from November 2022, re-introducing stations with real patients and examiners, while still retaining simulated retinoscopy. The format may be further changed in the future, so it is vital to get the most recent guidance from the Royal College of Ophthalmologists, which can be found online at www.rcophth.ac.uk/examinations/rcophth-exams/refraction-certificate/.

The College assesses competence in refraction using a multi-station objective structured clinical examination (OSCE). This is therefore a practical examination and candidates are not expected to be able to pass unless they have refracted many adults and children.

The examination assesses your ability in the following competencies that form part of the Ophthalmic Specialty Training (OST) curriculum:

- Assess vision and ocular motility
- Use spectacle lenses and prisms
- Perform a refractive assessment and provide an optical prescription
- Form management plan following assessment and investigations
- Establish good rapport with patient, using clear and concise communication
- Perform good hand hygiene
- Show effective time management
- Keep accurate clinical records
- Understand relevant optics and medical physics

DOI: 10.1201/9781003329329-2

Candidates are again examined on a number of different possible OSCE stations, so it is necessary to be competent in all of the following areas:

(1) Refraction of an adult
- History
- Trial frame fitting and interpupillary distance (IPD) measurement
- Visual acuity and refraction estimation
- Non-cycloplegic retinoscopy
- Subjective refraction of the sphere
- Subjective refraction of the cylinder
- Duochrome test and binocular balance
- Muscle balance with Maddox rod and prism cover test
- Near addition
(2) Refraction of a child
- Visual acuity testing in a child
- Cycloplegic retinoscopy
(3) Refraction of a model eye
(4) Establishing the prescription of a pair of spectacles
- Focimetry
- Lens neutralisation

The examination consists of multiple stations which could be examined in any number of different orders, but they are listed above in an order that makes clinical sense. For example, the stations listed under 'Refraction of an adult' are the steps typically taken to refract an adult in sequence from start to finish – which, once accomplished, typically should take 15 to 30 minutes.

The OSCE is composed of ten stations in total. There are five rooms, with two stations in each room. As of November 2022, two rooms (four stations) will require candidates to perform simulated retinoscopy on model eyes, while the remaining six stations can be any of those listed above. It is vital to become competent and comfortable in these skills, and this can only be achieved through consistent practice!

3

What does refractive error mean?

EMMETROPIA

'Emmetropia' means the absence of a refractive error, so parallel light from a distant source is perfectly focused on the retina (see Figure 3.1). An emmetrope will have normal distance acuity with no spectacles (uncorrected Snellen acuity of 6/6 or better) – provided, of course, there is no amblyopia, ocular pathology, or cerebral visual impairment.

REFRACTIVE ERROR (AMETROPIA)

'Refractive error' (ametropia) means that an eye does not allow light from a distant source to be focused perfectly on the retina. Approximately one-third of the population has a refractive error of more than 1 dioptre, and thus may need spectacles. Myopia is just as common as hypermetropia.

The refractive power of an eye is a function of the corneal curvature (accounting for two-thirds of the power; this can be altered through refractive surgery or specialty rigid contact lenses) and the crystalline lens (accounting for one-third of the power; this can be altered by accommodation, provided there is no presbyopia). This is a surprise to most people, since most assume that the crystalline lens is the most powerful refractive element. The air–cornea interface is in fact the most powerful refractive element – this becomes apparent when you dive into water without any goggles.

DOI: 10.1201/9781003329329-3

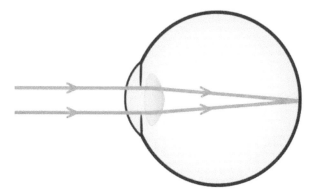

Figure 3.1 Emmetropia – light from a distant object forms an image on the retina

Refractive error (ametropia) occurs when the refractive power of the eye does not correspond optically with the axial length of the eye, so an image from a distant object does not fall on the retina.

Myopia

'Myopia' (short-sightedness) means that the refractive power of the eye is too great relative to the axial length of the eye; as a result, the image of a distant object lies in front of the retina (see Figure 3.2a). Therefore, myopia will result if the refractive power is too high or if the eye is too long. Myopia is corrected by a minus (concave) lens, which effectively weakens the refractive power to allow the image to be shifted back on to the retina (see Figure 3.2b).

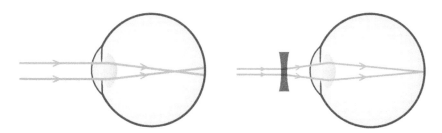

Figure 3.2 (a) Myopia – light from a distant object forms an image in front of the retina. (b) Myopia corrected by a minus (concave) lens which diverges rays

Hypermetropia

'Hypermetropia' (long-sightedness), also known as hyperopia, means that the refractive power of the eye is too weak relative to the axial length of the eye; as a result, the image of a distant object lies behind the retina (see Figure 3.3a). Therefore, hypermetropia will result if the refractive power is too low or if the eye is too short. Hypermetropia is corrected by a plus (convex) lens, which effectively strengthens the refractive power to allow the image to be shifted forwards on to the retina (see Figure 3.3b).

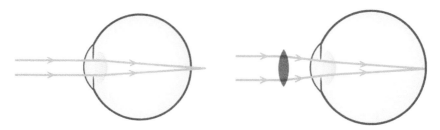

Figure 3.3 **(a)** Hypermetropia – light from a distant object forms an image behind the retina. **(b)** Hypermetropia corrected by a plus (convex) lens which converges rays

ASTIGMATISM

'Astigmatism' refers to the refractive power of the eye being different in different meridians. Therefore, light from a point of a distant object cannot form a single point of an image (see Figure 3.4).

An eye with astigmatism behaves as a sphero-cylindrical (toric) lens. The principal meridians form separate line foci and between them lies Sturm's conoid. The dioptric midpoint of Sturm's conoid is the circle of least confusion, situated at the focal point for the lens spherical equivalent value (see Figure 3.5).

The spherical equivalent of a sphero-cylindrical (toric) lens is equal to the sum of the sphere plus half the cyl, and is used to establish whether or not an eye with astigmatism can be considered overall to be myopic or hypermetropic (for more information, see section 'Notation, Transposition, and Spherical Equivalent').

This may sound quite complex, but basically, if an eye with astigmatism behaves as a sphero-cylindrical lens (i.e. a sphere lens with a cylindrical lens superimposed upon it), it follows that to correct astigmatism, a sphero-cylindrical lens is required. This is different to myopia or hypermetropia, which can simply be corrected with a spherical lens alone.

The origin of astigmatism is usually corneal, where the corneal curvature and, therefore, the refractive power are different in different meridians. This is why we often explain to patients that astigmatism implies that their eye is shaped like a rugby ball rather than a football.

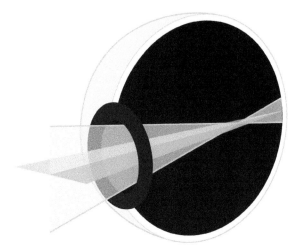

Figure 3.4 Astigmatism – light from the same distant point object does not form a single point image, as light is refracted by different amounts in different meridians

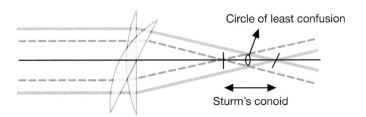

Circle of least confusion

Sturm's conoid

Figure 3.5 An eye with astigmatism behaves as a sphero-cylindrical lens, with the circle of confusion of Sturm's conoid lying at the focal point for the lens spherical equivalent value

The degree of corneal astigmatism can be assessed by a keratometer, which gives 'K' values for the refractive power in different meridians. The steeper the cornea in a given meridian, the greater the numerical value of the K value for that meridian.

If cataract surgery is proposed, it is important to consider the keratometer K values, since the site of the incision will flatten the cornea in this meridian. By placing the incision on the steepest K meridian, the degree of corneal astigmatism is reduced, which can be beneficial to the patient since astigmatism has no refractive advantage.

If astigmatism is present despite having a spherical cornea, it will be due to the crystalline lens (lenticular astigmatism). Lenticular astigmatism is eliminated by placing a spherical intra-ocular lens implant during cataract surgery. Some further terms used to describe astigmatism follow.

Regular astigmatism

This applies when the meridians of maximum and minimum refractive power are perpendicular to each other. This is further divided into:

'**with-the-rule**' regular astigmatism, in which:

- the steepest meridian is vertical, or within 30 degrees of 090 (060–120), and the flattest is horizontal (see Figure 3.6a, the steepest vertical meridian shaded grey)
- the maximal refractive power of the cornea acts vertically (the steepest K meridian will be near 090)
- the weakest refractive power of the cornea acts horizontally (the flattest K meridian will be near 180)
- the axis of a correcting plus cylinder will be vertical (090), since its power needs to act horizontally to strengthen the relatively weaker horizontal meridian
- An example of an eye that has with-the-rule regular astigmatism: +1.00 / +1.50 x 090. There is a +1.50 dioptre cyl, which has its axis (denoted by 'x') at 090. This cyl is superimposed on a +1.00 dioptre sphere. In the absence of any lenticular astigmatism, one would expect the K value in the vertical meridian to be greater than the horizontal meridian.

'**against-the-rule**' regular astigmatism, in which:

- The steepest meridian is horizontal, or within 30 degrees of 180 (000–030 and 150–180), and the flattest is vertical (see Figure 3.6b, the steepest horizontal meridian shaded grey)
- the maximal refractive power of the cornea acts horizontally (the steepest K meridian will be near 180)
- the weakest refractive power of the cornea acts vertically (the flattest K meridian will be near 090)
- the axis of a correcting plus cylinder will be horizontal (180), since its power needs to act vertically to strengthen the relatively weaker vertical meridian
- An example of an eye that has against-the-rule astigmatism: +2.00 / + 1.75 x 180. There is a +1.50 dioptre cyl with its axis (denoted by 'x') at 180. This cyl is superimposed on a +2.00 dioptre sphere. In the absence of any lenticular astigmatism, one would expect the K value in the horizontal meridian to be greater than the vertical meridian.

'**oblique**' regular astigmatism, in which:

- the maximal and minimal meridians are perpendicular to each other but are not acting at or within 30 degrees of the vertical or horizontal plane (see Figure 3.6c, the steepest meridian shaded grey)
  for example, a maximal meridian at 050 and a minimal meridian at 140.

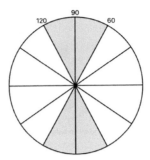

Figure 3.6a *With*-the-rule astigmatism

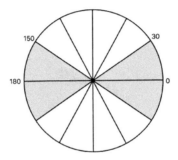

Figure 3.6b *Against*-the-rule astigmatism

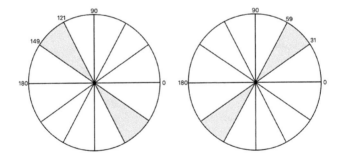

Figure 3.6c Oblique astigmatism

Irregular astigmatism

This applies when the meridians of maximum and minimum refractive power are not perpendicular to each other. The most common cause for this is keratoconus (which gives a scissor-like retinoscope reflex that is difficult to neutralise). Retinoscopy is of limited value for irregular astigmatism, and it is useful to map the corneal curvature more accurately with corneal topography. Irregular astigmatism is also common following corneal surgery such as 'penetrating keratoplasty' (full-thickness corneal graft).

Simple astigmatism

This is when the eye is plano (emmetropic) in one meridian (i.e. the rays in this meridian focus on the retina) and either myopic or hypermetropic in another (i.e. the rays in this meridian do not focus on the retina).

For example, 0.00 / +1.50 x 055 implies that no spherical correction is required, but a +1.50 cyl lens is required with an axis at 055 (power acting perpendicularly at 145) to correct the refractive error.

Compound astigmatism

This applies when both meridians are hypermetropic (i.e. the rays in all meridians come to focus behind the retina) or both are myopic (rays in all meridians come to focus in front of the retina).

For example, +1.00 / +2.00 x 090 implies that a +1.00 spherical lens with a +2.00 cyl lens with axis at 090 (power acting perpendicularly at 180) is required to correct the refractive error.

Mixed astigmatism

This applies when one meridian is myopic (rays fall in front of the retina) and the other is hypermetropic (rays fall behind the retina).

For example, −1.50 / +2.50 x 040 implies that a −1.50 spherical lens with a +2.50 cyl lens with axis at 040 (power acting perpendicularly at 130) is required to correct the refractive error.

NOTATION, TRANSPOSITION, AND SPHERICAL EQUIVALENT

A refractive error is expressed by the spectacle (or contact lens) prescription required to correct the refractive error in the form:

Refractive error = sphere/cyl x 000 (angle of cyl axis)

It is important to denote + or − for the sphere and the cyl value, and these values should be expressed to two decimal places (e.g. +0.75, −3.25). The angle of the cyl axis is expressed as a value from 000 to 180 (from right to left, anticlockwise, for either eye), and should always be three significant figures; the degree symbol should be omitted. For example, instead of writing '40°', write '040'.

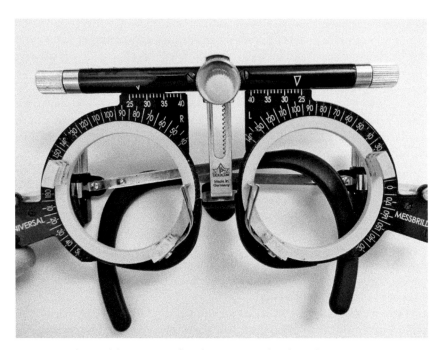

Figure 3.7 The trial frame provides demarcation for the cyl axis

If you get confused or cannot remember that the angle of the cyl axis runs from 000 to 180 from right to left (anticlockwise) for either eye, simply pick up a trial frame, as the angles are clearly demarcated on this (see Figure 3.7).

A spectacle prescription may be written in plus cyl notation or minus cyl notation – these are the two equivalent ways that any single refractive error can be corrected. Both plus and minus cyl notations are acceptable, so either can be used. Always ensure that for any single patient, both eyes are in the same notation (that is, both eyes in plus cyl notation or both eyes in minus cyl notation – never use plus cyl for one eye and minus cyl for the other eye). The notation that is chosen by someone usually reflects their training in retinoscopy. To obtain the equivalent notation, one form has to be transposed to the other form (transpose the plus cyl notation to the minus cyl notation, or vice versa).

Transposition involves three steps:
1 add the cyl to the sphere to give the new sphere
2 change the sign of the cyl to give the new cyl
3 the new axis is perpendicular to the old axis

Transposition example

Transpose –8.00 / +3.00 x 165.

New sphere = (–8.00) + (+3.00) = –5.00 (adding the cyl to the sphere to give new sphere)

New cyl = –3.00 (changing the sign of the cyl to give the new cyl)

New axis = 165 – 090 = 075 (the new axis is perpendicular to the old axis)

To give –5.00 / –3.00 x 075.

Therefore, –8.00 / +3.00 x 165 (plus cyl format) will correct the same refractive error as the transposed equivalent prescription –5.00 / –3.00 x 075 (minus cyl format).

It does not matter if you choose to record in plus or minus cyl notation, but it is crucial that you are consistent and for the eyes of any single patient, always use either plus cyl notation throughout for both eyes or minus cyl format throughout for both eyes. Do not use plus cyl for one eye and minus cyl for the other eye of the same patient, since such inconsistency is confusing and unacceptable in the Refraction Certificate examination.

Given that refractive prescriptions can be written in both plus or minus cyl format, it can be confusing at first to appreciate whether or not somebody is myopic or hypermetropic overall.

For example, consider –1.50 / +4.00 x 020, which is equivalent to +2.50 / –4.00 x 110. This person obviously has a significant amount of astigmatism, but are they myopic or hypermetropic overall? This can be simplified by the concept of the 'spherical equivalent', which corresponds to the circle of least confusion, and is the average refractive error of the two meridians of an individual eye, combining the effect of the sphere and cyl to decide if the eye is myopic or hypermetropic overall.

$$\text{Spherical equivalent} = \text{sphere} + (\text{cylinder}/2)$$

The spherical equivalent can be obtained from the refractive prescription in either the positive or the negative cyl format.

So, for the above example (–1.50 / +4.00 x 020 which is equivalent to +2.50 / –4.00 x 110), the spherical equivalent would be –1.50 + (+4.00 / 2) = +0.50. Note that this is equal to +2.50 + (–4.00/2) = + 0.50. The eye in this case can therefore be considered to, overall, be mildly hypermetropic.

This concept is particularly important to understand when choosing the intraocular lens power in cataract surgery, since if the incorrect target spherical equivalent is chosen, then anisometropia may result. 'Anisometropia' is when the difference in refractive prescriptions between the two eyes is sufficiently large to result in troublesome symptoms such as aniseikonia (different image size of single object between eyes) and asthenopia (eye strain – patients are often non-specific, but complain of fatigue, blurred vision, and headache).

This is different for different patients, but is a significant risk when the difference in spherical equivalent is more than 1.5 dioptres. It is therefore crucial to discuss with patients undergoing cataract surgery:

- Their target refraction (often the target is emmetropia, myopes often like to be left a little myopic, whereas there is no refractive advantage of being left hypermetropic unless this is done to avoid anisometropia in hypermetropic patients keen for cataract surgery in one eye only)
- The plan for the other eye (since a patient undergoing sequential, bilateral cataract surgery will often choose to be emmetropic but should be warned of anisometropia whilst awaiting second eye surgery).

4

How to refract

OVERVIEW

There are different ways to refract a patient (i.e. to obtain a spectacle prescription to correct refractive error). We detail a system that can be practised to correctly refract a patient and obtain all the necessary information required to complete the Refraction Certificate examination (at the time of writing).

Refracting a patient takes as long as it takes; however, the majority of cases can be refracted within 15 to 20 minutes. Practise is required and the system following provides a framework for this, which you can modify if necessary, according to the advice you are provided with whilst training. You will need to refract 70 to 100 patients before feeling comfortable with most situations and hence before you can pass the Refraction Certificate examination.

Remember that the certificate OSCE consists of multiple stations, so different parts of the refractive process may be examined in various orders. However, as already discussed, we have arranged these parts in an order that makes clinical sense. For example, the stations listed under 'Refraction of an adult' are those typically used to refract an adult in sequence from start to finish, which, as noted, typically takes 15 to 20 minutes.

Note that 'objective refraction' implies obtaining a refractive prescription that does not require any response from the patient – this is obtained by retinoscopy; for children or adults with learning disability, this may be the sole basis for a spectacle prescription. 'Subjective refraction' relates to fine-tuning the prescription obtained from retinoscopy by asking the patient a number of clear, closed questions whilst avoiding fatigue. This is where the art of refraction becomes evident!

The refractive process

The following is a useful template of the refractive process undertaken with an adult. Once experienced, it can take considerably less time, as the examination can be tailored to fit the patient; however, for the purpose of the Refraction Certificate examination, all components must be well rehearsed.

DOI: 10.1201/9781003329329-4

History (2 minutes)
IPD/trial frame/back vertex distance (1 minute)
Visual acuity (2 minutes)
Objective refraction – Retinoscopy (5–10 minutes)

- Typically without cycloplegia in an adult

Subjective refraction (5–10 minutes)

- Sphere
- Cyl axis
- Cyl power and sphere compensation
- Duochrome
- Binocular balance
- Maddox rod and prism cover test
- Near vision

Recording results (1 minute)

HISTORY

This should be brief – about 2 minutes. Introduce yourself, then ask the patient for their name and age. Clinically, it is useful to ask the following:

Do you wear spectacles or contact lenses?
Are your spectacles single vision, bifocal or varifocal?

- If bifocal or varifocal, presbyopia is relevant, so you will need a near add.

At what age did you start wearing spectacles?

- The younger the age, often the greater the refractive error and the higher the chance of amblyopia.

When do you wear your spectacles – when looking into the distance (such as when driving/watching television) or at things close by (e.g. when reading)?

- A mild myope may only wear them for distance.
- An emmetrope or mild hypermetrope who is older than 35 years (presbyopia may start to manifest from this point) may only wear them for reading.

Are you a driver?

- If so, their best corrected binocular visual acuity should be better than 6/ 12, which approximates the Driver and Vehicle Licensing Agency's legal requirement of being able to read a number plate with both eyes open at a distance of 20 metres away.

What is your occupation/hobby?

- Computer work may require a specific intermediate correction (a weaker near add to the distance prescription than that required for reading).

Do you do anything that requires you to see objects closer than at normal reading distance, such as sewing/model making?

- A stronger near add may be needed for such closer work.

Have you had any eye problems in the past?

- Has there been any surgery, laser, trauma, or drops?
- Have there been any problems with a lazy eye/use of patch as a child?
  - Amblyopia or previous eye disease may limit the best corrected visual acuity, so do not panic if 6/6 is not obtained in these cases.

Do you have any double vision – where you see two images?

- Patients may report blurred vision as double vision – always establish if two separate images are seen (true diplopia) and whether this is binocular (suggesting a squint without suppression) or monocular (suggesting unilateral ocular pathology such as a cataract, corneal scar, etc.).
- For binocular diplopia, it is important to assess the squint angle with the cover test and MR, and the patient may require prisms for their symptoms.

Inter-pupillary distance, trial frame, and back vertex distance

It should only take a minute or two to measure the inter-pupillary distance (IPD), fit the trial frame, and measure the back vertex distance (BVD).

Inter-pupillary distance

Explain to the patient that you are going to measure the distance between their pupils. Sit directly in front of them, resting a ruler on the bridge of their nose, ask the patient to look at your left eye and close your right eye. Line up the temporal limbus of the patient's right eye with the zero marking of your ruler. Ask them to look at your other eye (now close your left eye and open your right eye), and holding the rule very still, record the position of the nasal limbus of the left eye on the ruler in millimetres. The IPD typically lies between 55 and 75 mm.

Inter-pupillary distance near

Check you are at the same height as the patient and sitting level with the patient's reading distance. Ask the patient to look at the bridge of your nose. Close your right eye, and with your left eye, line up the zero of your ruler with the temporal limbus of the patient's right eye. Keeping your right eye shut, record the position of the nasal limbus of the patient's left eye on the ruler.

Typically, the IPD for near is 2 to 4 mm less than for distance due to the convergence that occurs with near stimulation.

Fit trial frame

Set your trial frame IPD to the distance IPD value you have just measured. Make the side arms as long as possible, then place on the frame on the patient's face, checking that the side arms hook around the ears and tighten the side arms until stable and comfortable. Check that the pupil is easily seen – if it is obscured in the horizontal plane, you will need to re-check your IPD; if it is obscured in the vertical plane, you will need to adjust the nasal rest (if the pupil is too high, lower the central frame bracket to elevate the trial frame; see Figure 4.1).

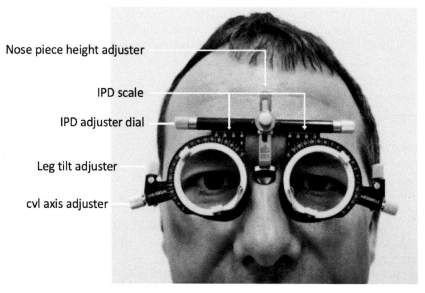

Nose piece height adjuster

IPD scale

IPD adjuster dial

Leg tilt adjuster

cvl axis adjuster

Figure 4.1 Correct fitting of a trial frame with each pupil in the centre of each aperture, both horizontally and vertically

Back vertex distance

Place a lens (of any value) in the trial frame. Ask the patient to fixate on a distant target, and use a rule to measure from the patient's cornea to the back of the lens (the surface of the lens nearest the cornea). A normal BVD is 12 to 14 mm.

The power of a lens system depends upon the distance of the lens from the cornea. This concept is known as 'lens effectivity' and explains why a myope's contact lens prescription will be numerically weaker than their spectacle prescription. It also explains why patients with powerful prescriptions get a blurred view when their spectacles slip down their nose.

Therefore, the BVD is important when a frame is to be constructed, since the function of the lens system depends not only on the lens power but also on the lens position relative to the cornea. Practically, this is relevant for prescriptions of more than 4 dioptres, but it is good practice to always record the BVD. Formulae exist to allow correction of any given prescription as well as BVD to a different prescription and BVD that will have an equivalent effect.

Visual acuity

'Acuity' is a measure of the resolving power of the eye – the ability to discriminate between two points. Distance charts that you should be comfortable with include the Snellen and the LogMAR. Near vision charts that you should be comfortable with include the N-series.

In any clinical setting, it is important to check the distance visual acuity for each eye (unaided, aided, and pinhole) and the near acuity for each eye (unaided and aided). If aided, it is useful to state if this is with spectacles or contact lenses. The eye not being tested should be correctly occluded.

For the purpose of the exam, the patient's spectacles will not be available, so the following will need to be established for each eye:

- distance acuity unaided (Snellen or LogMAR)
- distance acuity with pinhole
- near acuity unaided (N-series; remember to use a bright lamp).

Pinholes only allow axial rays through to the eye and hence reduce the effect of refractive error. Remember that the pinhole vision gives a good idea of potential vision for that eye once the refractive error has been corrected. Ideally, your target end-refraction visual acuity should be at least as good as the pinhole acuity. Remember that eyes with reduced pinhole vision or reduced vision despite adequate refractive correction have acuity that is limited by amblyopia, ocular pathology, or cerebral visual impairment. Pinhole acuity tends to partially improve with corneal or lens pathology but will not improve with amblyopia, retinal, nerve, or cerebral pathology (pinhole acuity can be worse than unaided acuity in patients with macular pathology, since it precludes eccentric fixation).

Always consider – why is the vision poor?

Refractive error:
. . . improves with pinhole.

Amblyopia:
. . . no improvement with pinhole.

Ocular pathology:
. . . if of retina or nerve origin, will not improve with pinhole.
. . . if of cornea or lens origin, may improve with pinhole.

Cerebral visual impairment:
. . . no improvement with pinhole.
Note, of course, a mixture of these reasons commonly coexists.

Refraction estimation

Checking the visual acuity will give you an idea of the refractive error:

- 1 dioptre of spherical error gives 6/12
- 2 dioptres of spherical error give 6/24 to 6/36
- 3 dioptres of spherical error give 6/60.

However, note that this guide is for spherical error and ignores that the patient may have astigmatism. The impairment in acuity is about half that for cylindrical errors relative to spherical errors. Therefore, a patient with 0.00 / +2.00 x 080 would be approximately 6/12 unaided.

This guide should only be used as an approximation, since patients will have a mixture of spherical and cylindrical errors.

This refraction estimation alone does not, however, suggest whether the patient is myopic or hypermetropic. For example, if they are 6/24 unaided, their refraction could be –1.75 or +1.75 spherical dioptres. To estimate if the patient is myopic or hypermetropic, compare their unaided distance acuity with their unaided near acuity. This concept is more useful if the patient is presbyopic, since otherwise the effect of accommodation confounds the estimation. If a patient has poor distance vision but good near vision, you know they are myopic. For example, if a presbyope has an unaided Snellen distance acuity of 6/60, yet is N5 at reading distance (on the near vision N-series reading chart), their refraction is probably around –2.00 to –3.00 spherical dioptres.

If they have poor distance vision and poor near vision, you know they are hypermetropic (or they have amblyopia, ocular pathology, or cerebral visual impairment – this should be clear from your history).

Visual acuity testing of a child

Although children can be unpredictable, which adds stress to an examination setting since it is something you cannot control, there are a number of useful ways of handling this that come with experience in assessing the visual behaviour of children.

It is important to spend time with orthoptic staff, since this is the best way to learn to be comfortable with the following:

- patching as a means of occlusion (note that objection to occlusion implies poor acuity in the other eye)
- assessing if a child's vision is central (i.e. no squint), steady (i.e. conjugate movements with no nystagmus) and maintained through the duration of a blink (i.e. there is sufficient acuity to fixate on and follow an object of interest, demonstrating that it is seen)
- preselected tests, such as Cardiff Cards, Kay Pictures, single optotype, or crowded charts, are used to assess binocular and monocular distance acuity.

RETINOSCOPY (OBJECTIVE REFRACTION)

Retinoscopy basics

The aim of retinoscopy is to obtain an objective refraction – that is, an estimation of the patient's spectacle prescription using a process that does not require any decisions to be made by the patient.

Retinoscopy also gives a good benchmark from which the prescription can be fine-tuned using subjective techniques (using subjective rather than objective refraction from the beginning takes considerably longer).

Retinoscopy is an invaluable process for children or adults with learning disability, as these patients will not be able to answer the questions required for subjective refraction. For these patients, your spectacle prescription will be based on your retinoscopy alone.

A retinoscope produces a light which, with the cuff fully down, is linear (the scope slit). For more information on the retinoscope, see Appendix 2. Quite simply, the scope slit light is passed across the patient's pupil and a light within the pupil (the reflex) is observed. By noting the quality of this reflex, various lenses are then placed in the trial frame to neutralise the reflex. As neutralisation is approached, the reflex will become faster and brighter. A dull, slow reflex implies neutralisation is not close. At neutralisation, the reflex is a glowing bright pupil; at this point, the lenses in the trial frame provide the objective spectacle prescription (once corrected for working distance).

The scope slit is held at a certain angle (say, vertically) and then swept across the pupil in a direction perpendicular to the orientation of the scope slit (in this case, horizontally). As the scope slit passes across the pupil, the reflex can be noted to have certain characteristics: (a) direction, (b) orientation, and (c) brightness and speed.

Characteristics of retinoscope reflex

Direction:

- with or against or neutralised

Orientation:

- vertical, horizontal, or oblique
- scissor reflex

Brightness and speed:

- bright and fast
- dull and slow

DIRECTION OF REFLEX

A 'with' reflex is seen if, as your slit passes across the pupil, a light within the pupil (the reflex) moves in the same direction (see Figure 4.2a). A plus lens must be added to the trial frame to approach neutralisation. An 'against' reflex is seen if, as your slit passes across the pupil, a light within the pupil (the reflex) moves in the opposite direction (see Figure 4.2b). A minus lens must be added to the trial frame to approach neutralisation.

To neutralise:

With reflex...add plus lens
Against reflex...add minus lens

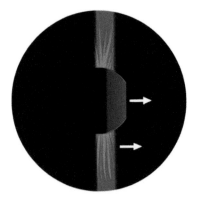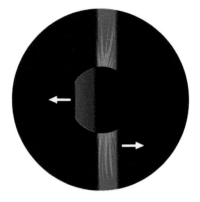

Figure 4.2 **(a)** A 'with' reflex. The scope slit is orientated vertically and swept horizontally across the pupil to give a with reflex. **(b)** An 'against' reflex. The scope slit is orientated vertically and swept horizontally across the pupil to give an against reflex

Therefore, to approach neutralisation, either a plus (if *with* reflex) or minus (if *against* reflex) must be added to the trial frame. If the reflex is already quite fast and bright, only 0.25 or 0.50 may be sufficient to reach neutralisation. To confirm neutralisation, you can lean backwards, further away from the patient (reflex becomes *against*) or lean forwards closer to the patient (reflex becomes *with*). This is because the closer you are, the more minus must be added to correct for the working distance (see section 'Correction for working distance'). Alternatively, to ensure the end point has been reached, add a +0.25 dioptre lens, which should give an *against* reflex. Such reversal of the reflex is important to achieve, since it highlights that the true end point of neutralisation has been established.

Note that the lenses added to approach neutralisation are either spherical or cylindrical. If a sphere is added to neutralise the reflex, it will also alter the subsequent lenses required in the perpendicular axis to obtain neutralisation. If a cylindrical lens is added (with the axis orientated the same way as the scope slit, so the power of the cylindrical lens will act in the same plane as the scope sweep), neutralisation in this plane is approached and has no effect on the other principal meridian.

ORIENTATION OF REFLEX

> The orientation of the retinoscope's slit light should be parallel to the pupil reflex.

If there is no astigmatism, or if the astigmatism is either with the rule or against the rule, the reflex will be orientated vertically and horizontally. In these situations, ensure the slit is vertical then horizontal (rotate the slit by rotating the cuff slightly) to neutralise these meridians.

With oblique astigmatism, the principal meridians are still perpendicular but do not strictly obey with the rule or against the rule. Therefore, when a horizontal scope sweep is made with the slit orientated vertically, the orientation of the pupil reflex will be oblique and not lie vertically. Similarly, if the scope slit was orientated horizontally and a sweep made vertically, the orientation of the pupil reflex will again be oblique and not be horizontal. For oblique astigmatism, the scope slit should be rotated by turning the cuff slightly so the slit is parallel to the pupil reflex to aid subsequent neutralisation (see Figure 4.3). The perpendicular meridian can then be neutralised by rotating the slit 90 degrees (e.g. if one meridian is at 130, the other will be at 40).

Another type of reflex is the 'scissor reflex', which occurs with a high degree of irregular corneal astigmatism, such as keratoconus. These reflexes can be difficult or simply not possible to neutralise. Keratoconus is a corneal ectasia, characterised by progressive stromal thinning and conical distortion, associated with increasing irregular astigmatism and myopia. It is appropriate to examine the eye on the slit lamp for other signs of keratoconus (stromal thinning/cone, Vogt's striae, Fleischer ring). Investigations include corneal topography so the degree of irregular astigmatism can be quantified and mapped. This aids the consideration of the various

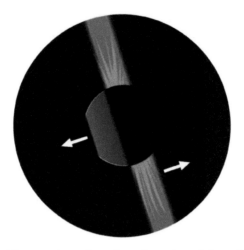

Figure 4.3 With oblique astigmatism, the orientation of the reflex will not be horizontal or vertical but oblique

available treatment options for keratoconus, including contact lenses, scleral contact lenses, or surgical intervention (riboflavin with ultraviolet A/collagen cross-linking, intra-stromal implants, deep lamellar or penetrating keratoplasty).

Brightness and speed of reflex

As mentioned, the brighter and faster the reflex, the closer to neutralisation. In these situations, use a small magnitude of lens power alteration (0.25 or 0.50 dioptres) since neutralisation is close. It's best not to get too bogged down to refine that extra + or –0.25, however, as you'll lose precious time, and induce accommodation in your patient.

Therefore, a dull, slow reflex is far from neutralisation and sometimes it pays to begin with a ±5 or ±10 dioptre spherical lens to start off with. Aphakia is a cause for high hypermetropia, with prescriptions of greater than +20 dioptres.

Remember, a dull reflex also occurs with medial opacity (such as with a cataract or vitreous haemorrhage). A dull reflex can also occur as a result of flat retinoscope batteries!

Correction for working distance

'Working distance' is the distance from the patient's cornea to your retinoscope. It is necessary to alter the sphere of the lenses in the trial frame to give a corrected full prescription based upon the value of the working distance.

The retinoscope is constructed so that if retinoscopy is performed at 1 m from the patient, the lenses in the trial frame to give neutralisation are equal to the spectacle prescription. However, we do not do retinoscopy at 1 m, but rather at 66 cm (when working with trial frames) or 50 cm (if you have shorter arms or when working without trial frames – for example, with children, examination under anaesthesia or a model eye).

Therefore, once neutralisation is obtained, to convert to the corrected prescription, it is necessary to add a –1.50 sphere to the trial frame (to correct for a 66 cm working distance) or a –2.00 sphere (to correct for a 50 cm working distance). Note that the cyl remains unchanged.

Therefore, a –1.50 myope will neutralise without any lenses if working at 66 cm. A –2.00 myope will neutralise without any lenses if working at 50 cm. Here are some other examples:

- neutralisation occurs with +4.25 / –1.75 x 030 at 66 cm, so the corrected refraction will be +2.75 / –1.75 x 030, since +4.25 plus –1.50 = +2.75
- neutralisation occurs with –3.75 / +0.75 x 044 at 50 cm, so the corrected refraction will be –5.75 / +0.75 x 044, since –3.75 plus –2.00 = –5.75.

Therefore, the working distance correction factor is the reciprocal of the working distance in metres, and this must be subtracted from the retinoscopy result.

Whenever a result is recorded, it is vital to state whether this is uncorrected or corrected for the working distance and what that working distance is. Therefore, add a –1.50 spherical lens for a working distance of 66 cm and add a –2.00 spherical lens for a working distance of 50 cm.

The correction of working distance can be done at the end of the retinoscopy once neutralisation has been achieved, whilst working at 66 cm or 50 cm. It can also be done at the start of retinoscopy. In this case, before using the retinoscope, you must add +1.50 (for 66 cm) or +2.00 (for 50 cm) to the trial frame (or your fingers, if working with no frame), and the resultant lens summation at neutralisation will give the corrected prescription. However, the answer forms will require you to write down your gross retinoscopy result, your working distance, and a corrected result accounting for your working distance.

Retinoscopy technique

Ideally, the room should be dim. The darker the room, the easier it is to note the reflex characteristics; if the room is too dark, you will struggle to find your lenses. A useful trick is to use your retinoscope light as a torch if you cannot see the lens markings easily. Ensure that your retinoscope has a divergent beam. This usually involves moving the cuff all the way down on the shaft of the retinoscope, but can be confirmed by shining the slit on a piece of paper – the slit should be wide and defocused.

> ## Key points for retinoscopy
>
> - Establish a dim room.
> - Fog (or occlude, if necessary) the fellow eye.
> - Scope the patient's right eye with your right eye/right hand.
> - Scope the patient's left eye with your left eye/left hand.
> - Keep your scope as close as possible to their visual axis, without interrupting continuous distant fixation.
> - Correct for working distance (add −1.50 sphere if at 66 cm; add −2.00 sphere if at 50 cm).
> - Record in either positive cyl notation for both eyes or negative cyl notation for both eyes (never positive for one eye and negative for the other).

The first step is to examine the patient's right eye with the retinoscope. For non-cycloplegic refraction of patients who are not presbyopic (especially if they are myopic), it is necessary to fog (blur) the fellow left eye. This involves placing a +1.50 or +2.00 spherical lens on top of the presumed refraction (estimated from their acuity, which you have just checked), so that the acuity is poorer than that of the eye being examined with the retinoscope.

Adequate fogging can be confirmed by ensuring that the retinoscopy reflex is against or, alternatively, checking the acuity in each eye with the fog in place and ensuring the fogged eye has poorer acuity than the eye about to be objectively refracted. If the patient is 6/6 with the presumed refraction, a +1.50 or +2.00 spherical dioptre fog typically renders the eye to 6/12 to 6/24.

The reason why the fellow eye should be fogged is to reduce accommodation, which would give a false result when examining the fellow eye with the retinoscope. With cycloplegic refraction (typically in children), there is no need to fog, since the accommodative component is removed by the cycloplegia. For non-cycloplegic refraction (most adults), fogging is required to reduce any accommodative drive (especially if the patient is a myope who is not yet presbyopic).

This fogging induces less accommodation than simple occlusion with a black occluder – hence, the effort made to fog rather than simply occlude.

Occlusion, rather than fogging, should be avoided, as it stimulates more accommodation. However, occlusion is required in the following situations:

- when the eye being tested is densely amblyopic (since the eye not being tested must have a poorer acuity to help avoid accommodation and a +2.00 lens will probably be insufficient to achieve this)
- if the patient markedly objects to fogging due to diplopia or asthenopia
- if you are unable to estimate acuity and provide an adequate fog lens.

Once you have adequately fogged (or, if necessary, occluded) the fellow eye, ask the patient to fixate on the white light or green target in the distance. Explain to them that it is important they continue to look into the distance and not at your

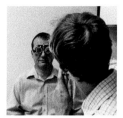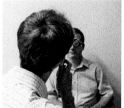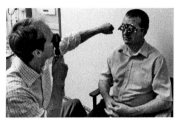

Figure 4.4 Examiner's working distance and head orientation during retinoscopy, without obscuring the patient's distant fixation target

own white light. Ask them to let you know if your head obscures their view of the distant fixation target. It is vital to ensure that your head is as close as possible to their visual axis, without actually obscuring their distant fixation target (see Figure 4.4) – this ensures that your retinoscope light will be close to their visual axis. Failure to be 'on axis' in this way can result in spurious astigmatism, so it is important to be wary of this when refracting children who shift their position.

Use your right hand and right eye to scope their right eye. Scope first with a vertical, then a horizontal, and finally a diagonal slit to locate the principal meridians. If only a dull, slow reflex is seen, try using a ±5 or even a ±10 dioptre lens. Then proceed by refracting in plus or minus cyls or spheres alone (see section 'Working in plus/minus cyls or spheres').

Once you have objectively refracted the right eye, correct for your working distance (add a –1.50 sphere if at 66 cm) and record your result. Then fog the right eye and use your left hand and left eye to scope their left eye. Once you have objectively refracted the left eye, again correct for working distance and record this. You should now turn the lights on, check the visual acuity and move onto subjective refraction.

Remember that if a *with* reflex is seen, then a plus lens (or less minus) should be added and if an *against* reflex is seen, then a minus lens (or less plus) should be added to approach neutralisation. The brighter and faster the reflex, the closer you are to neutralisation (the entire pupil lights up when the slit enters the pupil), whereas a dull and slow reflex implies you are not close to neutralisation.

Working in plus/minus cyls or spheres

It is possible to refract with your retinoscope in three different ways:

1 using positive cyls
2 using negative cyls
3 using spheres only

Generally, for those starting out with retinoscopy, identifying a *with* movement is easier to discern than *against*, and therefore using positive cyls is often preferred. The advantage of using negative cyls, and therefore favoured by more experienced practitioners, is that it induces less accommodation, since the spherical component is more positive.

Regardless of whether using positive or negative cyls, it is important to establish your principal meridians, and use the sphere component as your first meridian.

USING POSITIVE CYLS

This means that your retinoscopy result will be in a plus cyl format.

Identify the orientation of the two principal meridians, which will be perpendicular to each other. The principal meridian that has an *against* reflex – or, if both reflexes are *with*, it will be the least *with* reflex (which is fastest and brightest, as it is nearest neutralisation) – is neutralised first with spheres. This is the spherical component of your prescription. This will result in the other principal meridian giving a *with* reflex, which is then neutralised with positive cyls (the axis on the lens in the same orientation as the scope slit and pupillary reflex). The resultant prescription will be the lenses in the trial frame (which must then be corrected for working distance).

If when rotating from first to your second streak you see *against* instead of *with* motion, this is not a major error. It merely means the first meridian you found was not the sphere meridian. Keep your streak at its rotated orientation and reduce plus or increase minus to neutralise the *against* motion. This is the sphere meridian. Keep track of how much you had to change power because it will equal the power of the cylinder you need. Once neutralised, rotate your streak 90 degrees and you will see *with* motion. Neutralise this *with* motion with plus cylinder. The amount of power you had to change should equal the plus cylinder power you now use to achieve neutralisation.

For example, you identify an *against* reflex with scope slit at 135 and a *with* reflex at 045. Add minus spheres until the *against* reflex at 135 is neutralised (say, –3.00 causes neutralisation). Then add plus cyls (with the axis in the same orientation as the scope slit at 045) to neutralise the *with* reflex (say, +1.50 at 045 causes neutralisation). The axis line on the cyl lens should be parallel to the scope slit and light reflex (perpendicular to its power). The lenses in the trial frame then give the retinoscopy result in plus cyl format: –3.00 / +1.50 x 045, which must then be corrected for working distance (if at 66 cm, this gives –4.50 / +1.50 x 045).

This may sound complicated, but simply consider that a patient with regular astigmatism requires a sphere with a cyl superimposed upon it to correct their refractive error. The sphere is established first by neutralising the most *against* reflex, and the perpendicular meridian will then give a *with* reflex, which can be neutralised with plus cyls to give the sphero-cylindrical correction (which must be corrected for working distance).

USING NEGATIVE CYLS

This means that your retinoscopy result will be in a minus cyl format.

Identify the orientation of the two principal meridians, which will be perpendicular to each other. First, establish the spherical component by neutralising the most *with* reflex with plus spheres, then neutralise the perpendicular *against* reflex with minus cyls. The lenses in the trial frame will give the retinoscopy result in minus cyl format, which must then be corrected for working distance.

USING SPHERES ONLY

It is possible to obtain an objective refractive result without using any cylindrical lenses. Identify the two principal meridians. Neutralise one of the meridians with a sphere, record the result and orientation of reflex, then remove the sphere. Following this, neutralise the perpendicular meridian with a sphere and record the result and orientation of the reflex. The refractive result can then be expressed in either plus or minus cyl format; in both cases, the magnitude of the cyl is the difference between the two spheres. It can be useful to use a power cross to generate the resultant prescription.

Power crosses

As noted, if working in plus or minus cyls, the resultant refraction obtained by retinoscopy will simply be the lenses in the trial frame (this does not apply if working in spheres). This can then be corrected for working distance.

Therefore, it is not necessary to draw power crosses, and while power crosses are not required for the Refraction Certificate examination, they are an optional format of answer submission on the iPads used (at the time of writing). Furthermore, if you work only in spheres, it is useful to use a power cross to obtain your resultant refraction.

Each arrowed arm of a power cross represents the direction of movement of the retinoscope sweep. For example, when sweeping horizontally with the scope slit orientated vertically, the power in the horizontal plane (180) is examined. Therefore, if a sphere with power +3.50 dioptres neutralises a horizontal sweep, this implies the power in the horizontal direction is +3.50 dioptres. If a sphere with power +2.00 dioptres is then required to neutralise a vertical sweep with a horizontally orientated scope slit (to assess vertically acting power), the resultant power cross would be:

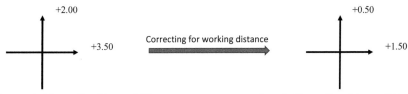

To obtain the prescription from the power cross in positive cyl notation:

- record the least positive meridian as the sphere
- record the cyl as the difference between the two meridians
- record the axis as the same axis of the most positive meridian (remembering that the axis is perpendicular to the direction of action of the power arrow)

The above example gives the prescription: +0.50 / +1.00 x 090, which when transposed, may also be written +1.50 / –1.00 x 180.

Here is another power cross example:

With slit at 045, power sweep at 135, a sphere of power –1.50 dioptres is required for neutralisation. With slit at 135, power sweep at 045, a sphere of power +0.25 dioptres is required for neutralisation. This gives the power cross:

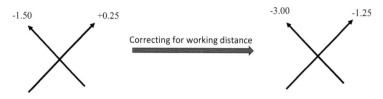

Which gives the prescription –3.00 / +1.75 x 135.

Interpreting the initial retinoscopy sweeps

When you are just starting, it is useful to have a clear idea in your mind of how to interpret the initial retinoscopy sweeps, since it is from here that you will make sequential decisions.

The level of your experience will become painfully obvious to the examiners at this early stage, so being confident and decisive at this point is a very good start.

It is useful to make three sweeps, one with the slit vertical, one horizontal, and then one that is obliquely orientated at a meridian that has become clear to you following the vertical and horizontal sweeps, if there is an oblique reflex.

Assuming you are working at 66 cm and have decided to work in plus cyls format, consider the seven possible initial scope sweep results:

(1) Neutralised in all meridians.
   The patient has a –1.50 ds refractive error.
(2) A dull, slow reflex that is difficult to interpret.
   Provided your battery has not been exhausted from all your enthusiastic work, the patient has a high degree of ametropia, so try interposing a + / – 5 or 10 lens. Remember, aphakia is a common cause of high hypermetropia, so don't mistake the initial dull, slow reflex for neutralisation!
(3) An *against* reflex in all meridians which is equally fast and bright.
   The patient is more myopic than –1.50 ds, and there is no significant astigmatism (neutralise with minus spheres).
(4) A *with* reflex in all meridians which is equally fast and bright.
   The patient is more plus than –1.50 ds, and there is no significant astigmatism (neutralise with plus spheres).
(5) An *against* reflex in one meridian, but more *against* (slower and duller) in another.

The patient has compound myopic astigmatism. Add minus spheres until the most *against* cyl is neutralised, leaving a perpendicular *with* reflex that can be neutralised with plus cyls.

(6) A *with* reflex in one meridian but more with (slower and duller) in another.

The patient has compound hypermetropic (or rather more plus than –1.50 ds) astigmatism. Add plus spheres until the least *with* cyl (faster and brighter reflex) is neutralised leaving a perpendicular *with* reflex that can be neutralised with plus cyls.

(7) A *with* reflex in one meridian and an *against* reflex in the perpendicular meridian.

The patient has mixed astigmatism. Add minus spheres to neutralise the *against* reflex, then add plus cyls to neutralise the *with* reflex.

Retinoscopy of a model eye

Practising retinoscopy on the model eyes, also known as the retinoscopy simulator, is helpful for several reasons. Firstly, at the time of writing, the Refraction Certificate examination requires candidates to perform simulated retinoscopy in four of the ten eyes of the exam, so it's well worth getting used to.

Secondly, the simulators are ideal for getting 'up and running' with objective retinoscopy in practice. The light reflex of the retinoscopy simulators is often easier to interpret than real reflexes; they avoid the need for cycloplegia, fogging of the fellow eye, or patient cooperation more generally, so practice can be performed in a relaxed and controlled environment on your own terms. Additionally, the retinoscopy simulator has a lens bracket and rotational adjustability of the dioptric power and pupillary diameter (see Figure 4.5). This means that with a trial lens set,

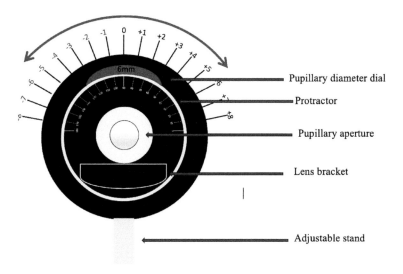

Figure 4.5 Illustration of the Heine retinoscopy simulator

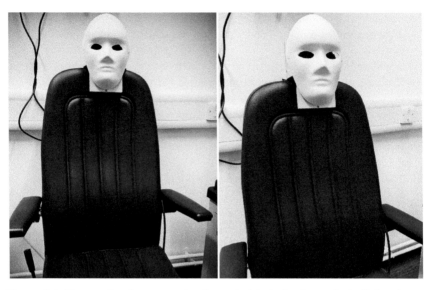

Figure 4.6 Mounted retinoscopy simulators behind plastic masks in Refraction Certificate examination station

a multitude of different prescriptions of varying complexity can be made up for a mock examination.

The Refraction Certificate examination uses the HEINE retinoscopy simulator, which is available in many trusts and at the Royal College of Ophthalmologists, but alternative and cheaper models are available to purchase online if access to HEINE simulators is limited.

The model eye is on an adjustable stand, however, the examination setting will be covered by a plastic mask and mounted on a chair, both to obscure the dioptric power setting and to mimic a real patient (see Figure 4.6). Since no trial frame can be used here, the practitioner needs to take care in judging their working distance and awareness of the cylindrical axis. This is a similar situation to performing retinoscopy on children (who are averse to trial frames), although in this case, there is no need to sing to the model eye in order to improve fixation!

If working in plus cyls, refract the model eye using spheres until the least *with* movement is neutralised, leaving a residual *with* movement in the perpendicular axis. Then, place a + cyl lens in front of the sphere (holding both lenses flush together) and rotate the cyl axis line so that it is orientated parallel to your scope slit. Continue to refract in this meridian until neutralised.

Great care must now be taken when recording your results. An approximation of the cyl axis must be made, since there is no trial frame to aid your recording of the cyl axis.

Furthermore, even if your working distance is typically 66 cm for refracting adults in trial frames, you'll probably find that your working distance for refracting children without trial frames (and therefore model eyes) is reduced to 50 cm. If your working distance is 50 cm, then it is necessary to add –2.00 ds to your prescription in order to correct for working distance (rather than the –1.50 ds which is added for a working distance of 66 cm).

Let's take a worked example:

In Figure 4.7, the dioptric power of the model has been set to 0 dioptres, and a +3.0 D cyl lens has been inserted into the lens bracket to simulate an eye with a sphero-cylindrical prescription. The +3.0 D cyl lens, with the axis at 180, will produce a myopic shift of 3.0 dioptres at 090 axis (think of the plus lens converging light to form an image before the retina in the vertical meridian). Assuming our working distance is 50 cm and that we are working in plus cyl, a horizontal slit swiping vertically will produce an initial *against* movement, and a *with* movement from a vertical slit swiping horizontally. The horizontal slit will be neutralised first with a –1.0 ds lens. Turning the slit perpendicular to the vertical, the horizontal meridian will be neutralised with an additional +3.0 cyl lens with the axis at 090, held flush against our –1.0 ds lens. Our gross prescription will be –1.0 / +3.0 x 090. Correcting for our working distance of 50 cm, we add –2.0 D to the sphere, producing a prescription of –3.0 / +3.0 x 090.

Alternatively, if working in spheres, the vertical meridian will be neutralised with a –1.0 ds lens, and the horizontal meridian with a +2.0 ds lens. The same gross and corrected prescription for working distance will be produced as above.

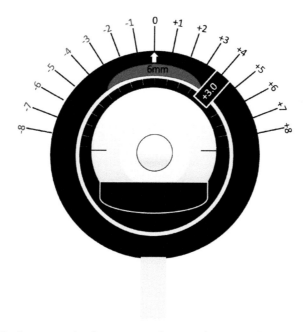

Figure 4.7 Retinoscopy simulator set to plano, with +3.0 cyl lens in the lens bracket, axis at 180

The simulator dioptric power setting can be altered to myopic or negative prescriptions, superimposed with cyl lenses placed in the lens bracket, with the axis at varying degrees, to mimic more complex compound and mixed astigmatism that can be with-/against the rule/oblique.

Cycloplegic versus non-cycloplegic retinoscopy

'Cycloplegia' refers to paralysis of the ciliary muscle, so that accommodation is not possible. Cycloplegics, such as topical cyclopentolate, will cause mydriasis (pupil dilatation) in addition to cycloplegia.

Non-cycloplegic retinoscopy is often sufficient for the majority of adult patients, especially if they are presbyopic (no effective accommodation). However, in the following situations, it is useful to perform cycloplegic refraction:

- in children and young adults (especially if they are myopic) to remove accommodation, which gives a falsely myopic refraction if not removed
- in adults with small pupils or opaque media (such as a corneal scar or cataract) who have a poor-quality retinoscopic reflex without pupil dilatation

Ensure that cycloplegia is complete by instilling the cycloplegic and waiting at least 30 minutes. Check that there is no miosis following illumination of the pupil. Since cyclopentolate can sting, consider first giving a topical anaesthetic for children. Note that the pupil dilatation occurs before the full cycloplegic effect, so it is necessary to wait the full 30 minutes, even if the pupil is dilated after 10 minutes.

OTHER ASPECTS OF CYCLOPLEGIC RETINOSCOPY

- If the patient is a child (or an adult with learning disability), trial frames are not always tolerated. Try half-aperture child trial frames or simply hold the lens in front of each eye in turn.
- Children are less likely to remain still. The challenge here is to ensure your retinoscope light is on the visual axis of the child, since spurious astigmatism is noted if you are not co-axial to the eye. It is also harder to keep a constant working distance, which is typically shorter for a child (50 cm, with a –2.00 dioptre working distance correction) than for an adult (66 cm, with a –1.50 dioptre working distance correction).
- Neutralisation can be harder to appreciate. The direction of the initial retinoscopic reflex can be easier to determine in dilated eyes, but this can give a false sense of security, as the neutralisation point can be more difficult to establish. It may seem that neutralisation occurs over a wider range of lenses relative to non-cycloplegic refraction – it is important to watch the central reflex of the dilated pupil and 'push' the lenses until clear reversal is seen. For example, neutralisation may seem to occur at +2.00 dioptres, but do not settle for this – *push the plus*. It will then become apparent, for example, that the central reflex gives a better neutralisation reflex at +3.00 dioptres and reversal is seen with +3.25 dioptres.

- Accommodation is not active – there is no need for the patient to comply with distant fixation and there is no need to fog the fellow eye.

OTHER ASPECTS OF NON-CYCLOPLEGIC RETINOSCOPY

- Trial frames are typically tolerated in adult non-cycloplegic retinoscopy, and these can help with establishing a more accurate angle of an astigmatic meridian.
- Patients are generally still. This makes it easier for your retinoscope's light to remain co-axial with the patient's eye, thus reducing the risk of spurious astigmatism.
- With small pupils or opaque media (such as a corneal scar or cataract), the reflex can be difficult to interpret. A dim room will dilate the pupil and help with this.
- Accommodation is active in pre-presbyopes (especially if myopic); this can be reduced by fogging the fellow eye adequately, maintaining distant fixation and avoiding prolonged retinoscopy bursts (try to decide within the first couple of sweeps and always within a few seconds).

Reducing accommodation in non-cycloplegic retinoscopy:

1. fog fellow eye
2. ensure the patient maintains distant fixation
3. avoid prolonged retinoscopy bursts

Failure to reduce accommodation gives a spuriously myopic result.

Finally, some important retinoscopy tips:

- Keep your lenses tidy (it will infuriate the examiners having to tidy up after you, and it's unfair on the candidates entering the station after you).
- Put your next lens into the trial frame before taking a lens out (this will minimise accommodation).
- No retinoscopy sweep should last more than a few seconds. Prolonged sweeps not only induce accommodation (if non-cycloplegic) but also demonstrate to the examiners that you do not know how to act in response to what you see. Therefore, if you are not sure after a few seconds, come away, put a different lens in and try again.
- If the reflex is too dull to interpret, check your retinoscope battery. If the battery is OK, you are dealing with high ametropia. Try interposing a ±5 or ±10 sphere.
- If the results are too minus, check that the patient is not accommodating, either because they are not looking at the distant target (patients need constant

reminders to do this) or because you have occluded rather than fogged the fellow eye. Occlude the fellow eye when checking visual acuity, but when using your retinoscope and for subjective refraction fog the fellow eye (with a +2 to + 4 add on your estimated prescription to reduce accommodation). If the patient is amblyopic or diplopic, avoid fogging and simply occlude the fellow eye for retinoscopy and subjective refraction. If accommodation is an issue (as it is with all children), cycloplegic refraction is required.

- If the results are too plus, remember to subtract the working distance correction factor.

Subjective refraction

Subjective refraction involves the patient making conscious decisions so that a prescription that has been approximated by objective means (retinoscopy) can be fine-tuned.

Therefore, this is not always possible in children or patients with learning disability, so your retinoscopy result will provide the basis for spectacle prescription in these patients.

The aim is not to under-correct myopia nor overcorrect hypermetropia, which will otherwise induce accommodation.

The process of subjective refraction should start within 10 minutes of the refractive process and take no longer than 10 minutes. The process includes the following stages:

1. refining the sphere
2. refining the cyl axis
3. refining the cyl power with sphere compensation
4. duochrome testing
5. binocular balance testing
6. MR and PCT
7. near vision testing

The refinement of the sphere and cyl and duochrome test is completed first for the right eye and then for the left eye.

Binocular balance is then tested with both eyes open.

The MR test (and possibly PCT) is used to assess the tendency of the eyes to dissociate, and to establish if prisms are required to control a symptomatic tropia.

Following this, the near vision is corrected and tested with appropriate correction for the right and then the left eye (test each eye independently).

Retinoscopy should be conducted in dim light. Subjective refraction should be conducted in good light – so when you put your retinoscope down, turn the lights back on.

Ensure you have recorded your retinoscopy results (corrected for working distance) and the visual acuity that was obtained with these.

As with retinoscopy, during subjective refraction, it remains important to fog the fellow eye (or, if appropriate, occlude the fellow eye). This not only reduces accommodation in non-cycloplegic refraction but also ensures that the patient's answers to your subjective refraction questions are based entirely on the eye being examined.

In addition, as with retinoscopy, when changing a lens, always put the next lens into the trial frame before taking a lens out, to minimise accommodation.

Refining the sphere

Ask the patient to fixate on one of the letters on the lowest line of the acuity chart that they can see comfortably.

Ask the patient:

Is that letter clearer with [place a +0.25 sphere in front of their eye] *or without the lens* [remove the +0.25 sphere] *or about the same?*

If a response is not immediately given, after only a couple of seconds, remove the lens, wait a couple of seconds, then re-offer them the lens and repeat the question. Do not simply hold the lens up waiting for a decision, since the quality of the answer diminishes rapidly with time. If no response is succinctly given, it is likely that the letter remains about the same.

If the patient reports that the letter is better or about the same, add the plus lens to the frame and repeat.

If they report that the letter is worse with the plus lens, do not give the plus lens. Instead, offer them a −0.25 sphere and ask them:

Is that letter better, or just smaller and darker?

This minus lens should only be offered for a brief moment to avoid accommodation. If they immediately report that the letter is better, add the −0.25 sphere to the trial frame and repeat. If they report that the letter is smaller and darker, check the acuity and move onto refining the cyl. If they report that the letter is worse (even though you did not ask them this), check the acuity and move onto refining the cyl.

Noticing that a letter is smaller and darker rather than actually better can be difficult, and there is the danger of overcorrecting accommodating myopes. Therefore, be slightly reluctant to keep giving minus spheres to a myope (such experience comes with practise).

Note that when the −0.25 sphere is offered, only hold this up for a couple of seconds. If the patient does not make a decision quickly, remove the −0.25 sphere and re-offer them the lens and the question. Do not simply hold the lens up waiting for a decision, since the quality of the decision will decrease with time and, in the case of this minus lens, the patient will accommodate.

Using a ±0.25 sphere to refine the sphere is appropriate if the acuity is 6/9 or better. If the acuity is between 6/12 and 6/18, use a ±0.50 sphere, and consider using a ±1.00 sphere if it is worse than 6/18.

To avoid inducing accommodation:

When adding a plus lens: for hypermetropes, do not remove the lens from the trial frame before adding the new lens. For myopes, remove the original lens before adding the new lens

Only add a minus lens to a myope if it makes the vision better, rather than just smaller and darker

At this stage, do not panic if the acuity is poor and cannot be improved. It may be that the patient has a large cyl (a high degree of astigmatism). Therefore, move onto refining the cyl when an end point is reached, rather than persevering only with spheres in the pursuit of perfect acuity.

Refining the cyl axis

Refining the cyl follows refining the sphere. The fogging of the fellow eye should remain in place and, for the purpose of the Refraction Certificate examination, if demonstrating subjective refraction of the cylinder only, adequate fogging must first be ensured.

The cylindrical component of the spectacle prescription is fine-tuned subjectively using the Jackson cross cylinder (JCC), which was first described by Edward Jackson in 1887.

The JCC is a sphero-cylindrical (toric) lens in which the power of the cylinder is twice the power of the sphere and of the opposite sign. The JCC is equivalent to superimposing two cylindrical lenses of equal power but opposite sign with their axes perpendicular to each other. The handle of the JCC is 45 degrees to the axes of the cyls. Since there are two perpendicular opposing cyls, an axis for the JCC is not denoted. The spherical equivalent (equal to the sphere plus half the cyl) of a JCC is therefore zero.

If a −0.25 cyl is superimposed perpendicularly with a +0.25 cyl, the net result is equivalent to −0.25/+0.50 (when transposed equivalent to +0.25/−0.50). This would be a 0.50 JCC, since the JCC is defined by the power of the cyl notation.

JCCs are available in various powers, typically 0.50 and 1.00, and this is usually written on the shaft (see Figures 4.8 and 4.9). The power is named after the power of the cyl given by its notation. Hence a −0.25 / +0.50 (same as +0.25 / −0.50) is a 0.50 JCC and a −0.50 / +1.00 (same as +0.50 / −1.00) is a 1.00 JCC. The 0.50 JCC is used if acuity is 6/12 or better, whereas the 1.00 JCC is used if acuity is worse than 6/12.

Do not rely on the colour of the JCC axes to confirm which is plus and which is minus – the only way to be sure is to look at the lens markings. A 0.50 JCC will have +0.25 written on the lens and, perpendicular to this, −0.25 will be denoted. A 1.00 JCC will have +0.50 written on the lens and, perpendicular to this, −0.50 will be denoted. It should be acceptable to take your own JCCs to the examination if you wish.

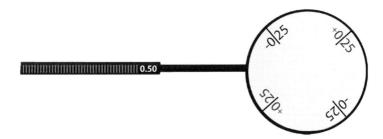

Figure 4.8 A 0.50 JCC (–0.25 / +0.50)

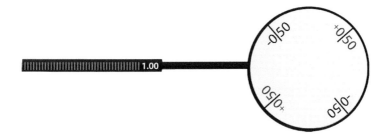

Figure 4.9 A 1.00 JCC (–0.50 / +1.00)

To check the cyl axis (established by retinoscopy) with the JCC, hold the handle along the proposed plus axis. Ask the patient to look at the letter O (or other types of circular targets such as two double rings).

Ask them:

Does the O look rounder and clearer with lens 1 [position 1 – handle along axis] *or lens 2* [position 2 – twist 180 degrees] *or about the same?*

Note that this question forces a comparison between the JCC in position 1 and the JCC position 2, *not* a comparison without the JCC. If the patient reports that both are equally bad, this should be interpreted as meaning that position 1 is the same as position 2.

When working in plus cyls, if the patient prefers position 1, rotate the cyl so the axis moves towards the plus cyl of the JCC when in position 1. If the patient prefers position 2, rotate the cyl so the axis moves towards the plus cyl of the JCC when in position 2.

The amount of rotation required (range 2 to 20 degrees in any alteration) depends upon the acuity and the strength of the cyl. If acuity is already good, only move the cyl by small amounts to avoid losing the good acuity. If the cyl is large, avoid large movements, since only a couple of degrees of movement of a large cyl can make quite a difference. This appreciation comes with practice. If unsure, apply the 'bracketing' technique, in which you initially move the axis by 20 degrees, then re-check and move by 10 degrees, then 5 degrees, then 2 degrees to reach the desired end point. Never underestimate the importance of obtaining the correct axis for a high-powered cyl.

If the patient reports that position 1 is the same as position 2 (or, as is quite common, appears to reject both of them), an end point has been reached and a satisfactory axis has been obtained. Now move onto refining the cyl power.

Refining the cyl power with sphere compensation

Ask the patient to focus again on the distant circular target.

When working in plus cyls, hold the *plus JCC axis over the plus cyl axis in the trial frame* (position 3 – this increases the cyl power).

Ask the patient to:

Look at the O – does the O look rounder and clearer with lens 3 [position 3] *or lens 4* [position 4 – twist 180 degrees, this places the minus JCC axis over the plus cyl axis in the trial frame to decrease the cyl power] *or about the same?*

Again, the forced comparison is between the two positions of the cross cyl, and not a comparison with no cross cyl.

If position 3 is preferred, add +0.50 cyl to the plus cyl and add –0.25 sphere. This *sphere compensation* when adjusting the cyl ensures the spherical equivalent of the lenses is maintained (spherical equivalent = sphere + cyl/2). To maintain the spherical equivalent, the sphere must be changed by half the amount of the cyl and in the opposite direction.

If position 4 is preferred, reduce the plus cyl power by 0.50 cyl and add +0.25 sphere to maintain the same spherical equivalent.

If the cyl power is changed (and sphere compensated), it is necessary to re-check the axis and challenge the cyl power again. If you do not trust the cyl obtained, reduce the cyl (or remove if small) and see if the patient prefers this (i.e. test for rejection of cyl), since patients are more likely to prefer under- rather than over-astigmatic correction.

Continue this process until an *end point* is reached for both the cyl axis and cyl power (i.e. until the patient reports that position 1 is same as 2, and position 3 is the same as 4).

Re-check the acuity, then proceed to the duochrome test.

Duochrome test

This is a monocular subjective test to minimise accommodation whilst the distance prescription is worn, which is especially important in myopes.

If a myope is overcorrected (prescription too minus), they are effectively rendered hypermetropic and may experience asthenopia (eye strain) due to prolonged accommodation.

The principle of the duochrome test relies on chromatic aberration, which is where white light, when refracted at an optical interface, is dispersed into its different colours (wavelengths).

An emmetropic eye focuses distant yellow–green light (555 nm wavelength) perfectly onto the retina. Red and green light are used for the duochrome, since their wavelength foci straddle yellow–green light by equal amounts (about 0.4 dioptres on either side), with green being deviated more than red, since red has the longer wavelength (see Figure 4.10).

The duochrome consists of a ring of black circles or letters on a red and green background (see Figure 4.11).

After the JCC test, whilst the fellow eye is still fogged, ask the patient to look at the distant duochrome and ask if the circles/letters are clearer on the red, green, or about the same. If they prefer green, add +0.25 sphere and repeat the question. Adding plus spheres should shift the preference from green to indifferent to red, and should relieve any accommodation with sacrificing the acuity.

Most practitioners would agree to leave myopes just on the red. For myopes, green is generally considered unacceptable, indifference (equal red and green) acceptable, and just on the red preferable. The reason why myopes should not be left on the green is that they will be accommodating, as the prescription is too minus (i.e. overcorrected, rendering them hypermetropic).

This test is less important for hypermetropes – leave them indifferent or just on the green. Note that the test can also be done in patients who are colour blind, since the test is dependent on the position of the image with respect to the retina.

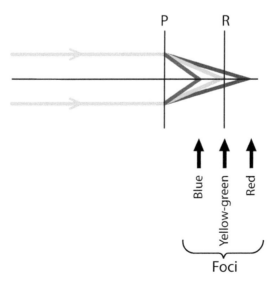

Figure 4.10 Dispersion and the human eye. Yellow–green light (555 nm) is focused perfectly onto the retina (R) by an emmetropic eye, when light is dispersed by the principal plane (P) of the optical interface. Blue light falls in front of the retina and red light falls behind the retina by equal amounts

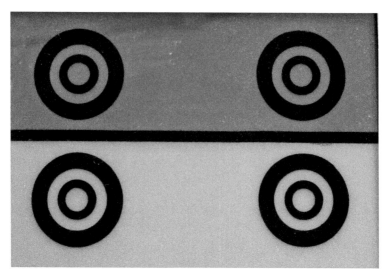

Figure 4.11 The duochrome

Therefore, colour-blind patients can be asked if the left or right (or upper or lower) rank is clearer, rather than the red or green rank.

Once adjusted, re-check the acuity.

As an extra step in myopes, it is useful to try the +1.00 blur back test, in which a +1.00 sphere is added that should blur the acuity to 6/12. If the myope remains 6/6, the prescription is too minus (overcorrected) and this +1.00 spherical lens should be added to their prescription to remove their accommodation, whilst retaining distance acuity.

The duochrome test is then repeated for the left eye (remember to fog the right eye).

Binocular balance

This is a final step to balance any accommodation and is done once both eyes have been independently subjectively refracted. It is particularly useful in young myopes to ensure that their prescription is not too minus (overcorrected) and is an alternative to the +1.00 blur back test already described (see above).

Check the binocular acuity (remove any fogging or occluding lenses).

Now ask the patient to fixate on a letter on the lowest line that they can see.

Then place a +1.00 sphere over the left eye and a +0.25 sphere over the right eye and ask:

Is the letter better, worse, or about the same?

If the letter is better or about the same, add the +0.25 sphere to the right eye and repeat. Do not give the plus lens if the letter appears worse (blurred).

Repeat the process with the +1.00 sphere over the right eye and the +0.25 sphere over the left eye.

If any lenses are added, re-check the binocular acuity to ensure that it has not reduced. If acuity has fallen, remove the plus lens.

COVER AND ALTERNATE COVER TESTS

These tests are useful in assessing the angle of deviation in eyes that have a squint or a tendency to drift.

It is important to understand these, since they are very quick to perform and often yield invaluable information. They also form a basic standpoint from which the PCT or MR test progresses so that the squint can be quantified with prisms and prismatic incorporation can be considered in the spectacle prescription for significantly symptomatic patients.

Cover test

This is a quick test that is used to detect a manifest squint (tropia).

Remember that children (or adults with untreated childhood squint) with a manifest squint will suppress the image from the weaker, non-fixating eye and therefore not complain of diplopia. In contrast, adults with a recently acquired squint will complain of binocular diplopia that is worse when they look *in the direction* of extra-ocular muscle under-action.

The cover test should be performed:

- with and without spectacles
- with and without any compensatory head posture
- for distance and near (to torchlight and an accommodative target)
- always in the primary position and, if necessary, in the different directions of gaze

For the distance cover test, ask the patient to fixate on a distant (6 m) target. Remember to first gently guide the patient's head into the primary position to remove any compensatory head posture.

Cover the left eye and observe for any movement in the right eye (see Figure 4.12).

- Esotropia (convergent squint) when the right eye initially is pointing nasally and then moves temporally on cover test.
- Exotropia (divergent squint) when the right eye initially is pointing temporally and then moves nasally on cover test.
- Right hyper-/hypotropia (vertical squint) when the right eye initially is higher/lower than the left and then moves downwards/upwards on cover test.

Now repeat the cover test with the right eye occluded, observing the movement of the left.

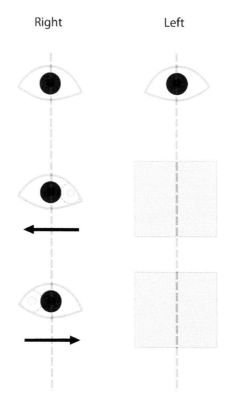

Figure 4.12 The cover test demonstrating a right esotropia (middle picture) and exotropia (bottom picture)

If there was movement with left eye occlusion but not for right eye occlusion, the tropia will be a 'right eye' tropia (e.g. right esotropia if the right eye moved temporally), since the left eye is the more stable eye that is adopting fixation (and vice versa for movement with right eye occlusion but not left eye occlusion). Repeat the cover test with spectacles and with any compensatory head posture. Then repeat the cover test with a near torchlight followed by a near accommodative target, such as a small attention holding image at 33 cm (reading distance).

Alternate cover test

The alternate cover test is a dissociative test that dissociates, or uncouples, the eyes. As each eye 'sees' a different fixation target, their true tendency to drift is released. As the alternate cover test continues, this tendency to drift often becomes more marked.

Therefore, the amount of deviation noted with the alternate cover test is the sum of both the manifest squint (detected with the cover test) and the latent component of the squint (the tendency of the eyes to drift once dissociated). If the deviation is observed with the cover test alone, this is known as a '-tropia'. If there is no deviation with the cover test but there is with the alternate cover test, this isolated latent component is known as a '-phoria'.

As with the cover test, the alternate cover test should be performed:

- with and without spectacles
- with and without any compensatory head posture
- for distance and near (to torchlight and an accommodative target)
- always in the primary position and, if necessary, in the different directions of gaze

For the distance alternate cover test, ask the patient to fixate on a distant (6 m) target. Remember to first gently guide the patient's head into the primary position to remove any compensatory head posture.

Cover the left eye and observe for any movement in the right eye. Then swiftly move the occluder to cover the right eye and observe for any movement as the left eye becomes uncovered. Repeat this a few times until the degree of movement has settled (since it will increase with time) and once you have noted the direction of movement.

- A temporal movement (from initial nasal, convergent position) implies an esodeviation.
- A nasal movement (from an initial temporal, divergent position) implies an exodeviation.
- A down/up movement (from an initial high/low position) implies a hyper-/ hypo- (vertical) deviation.

If the eyes rapidly take up fixation, then this suggests the acuity and subsequent neural link with the visual pathways are similar for each eye. If one eye is slow to take up fixation (sometimes requiring verbal encouragement), it is likely that the acuity in this eye is poor.

Repeat the alternate cover test for near torchlight, then a near accommodative target at 33 cm reading distance.

Prism cover test

The PCT allows the measurement of the angle of deviation, which allows objective quantification of the squint and subsequent prescription of the prism for symptomatic control if necessary.

As with the cover test, the PCT should be performed:

- with and without spectacles
- with and without any compensatory head posture
- for distance and near (the patient can hold the near accommodative target)
- always in the primary position and, if necessary, in the different directions of gaze

Note that the PCT should be performed for distant and near accommodative targets and different prisms may be required for distance and near prescriptions, since patients tend to converge on near fixation. Since the examiner requires one hand to hold the prism bar and one hand to move the occluder, when testing the angle for a near accommodative target, it is necessary to ask the patient to hold, and look at, the accommodative target.

A prism can be held in front of either eye, since the angle of deviation relates to the angle between the eyes. If you are right-handed, you may find it easier to hold the occluder in your left hand and the prisms in your right hand. The prisms can be held individually or in the form of a prism bar – whichever you feel more comfortable with.

A combination of horizontal and vertical prisms may be needed. First, establish and neutralise the horizontal angle, since these are usually larger. Once this is corrected, look specifically for a vertical deviation and superimpose vertical prisms on the horizontal prism to correct the vertical component.

Vertical deviations are typically smaller than horizontal deviations, but in the absence of suppression (such as with an acquired squint in an adult in the case of thyroid eye disease or cranial nerve 4 palsy), they are often more symptomatic due to the binocular fusion range being smaller vertically rather than horizontally.

Note that prisms will have a form of demarcation, such as a cross, at their base to help orientation.

For the distance PCT, ask the patient to fixate on a distant (6 m) target. Remember to first gently guide the patient's head into the primary position to remove any compensatory head posture.

Perform an alternate cover test as described.

Repeat the alternate cover test with a prism in place:

- for exodeviations, a base-in (BI) prism is needed
- for esodeviations, a base-out (BO) prism is needed
- for hyper-/hypodeviations, a BD/BU prism is needed.

There is no need to remember these listed points – just remember that *the correcting prism must have its apex pointing in the direction of deviation.*

If the movement is in the same direction with this corrective prism, the strength of the prism must be increased. If the movement has reversed direction, the prism strength must be reduced. The aim is to alter the prisms until reversal is noted, to obtain a satisfactory *end point*, which is when the eyes remain still during the alternate cover test since the prisms have neutralised any deviation. This can be confirmed by asking the patient if their double vision has been eliminated.

As mentioned, first correct the horizontal angle, then look specifically for a vertical component and correct this, if present, by superimposing vertical prisms upon the correcting horizontal prism.

Now repeat the test for a near accommodative target (held by the patient at 33 cm reading distance). The patient should wear their near spectacles (albeit without prisms at this stage).

When incorporating prisms into the spectacle prescription, the term 'prism dioptre' can be denoted by a triangle (Δ). However, as this can be mistaken for a zero, it is safer to use the abbreviation 'pd' in the spectacle prescription. The amount of deviation in degrees is corrected by a prism with a power double that magnitude in prism dioptres. For example, a 15-degree angle of deviation is corrected by a 30 pd prism.

Typically, the prismatic correction is halved between the two lenses and the bases will be in the same direction for horizontal deviations and in opposite directions for vertical deviations. For example, a 13 pd exodeviation will be corrected by a 6 pd BI correction in front of the right eye and a 7 pd BI correction in front of the left eye. A 4 pd right hyperdeviation will be corrected by a 2 pd BD correction in front of the right eye and a 2 pd BU correction in front of the left eye.

> Remember that the apex of the correcting prism is always in the direction of squint deviation.

Maddox rod

The Maddox rod (MR) test is a subjective assessment of extra-ocular muscle balance, and estimates the degree of phoria (tendency of eyes to drift so they are not directed at the same target), which can then be corrected by incorporating prisms into the spectacle prescription.

The majority of patients do not need prisms. Prisms should only be incorporated into the spectacle prescription if

- there is a history of double vision, or significant asthenopic (eye strain) symptoms
- if a manifest squint (tropia) is noticed with the cover test
- restoration of orthophoria is achieved with the proposed prisms using the MR test (and prism cover test)

If there is no double vision and if no tropia is seen with a cover test, then the MR test is academic since regardless of what it shows, there will be no need for prismatic correction. Therefore, in the Refraction Examination, always consider that the correct answer is in fact to order no prisms.

You may find that some patients without any refractive correction have acuity that is too poor to allow them to appreciate multiple images. Without their spectacles, they do not complain of diplopia since everything is simply blurred. In these cases, you will notice that once you have improved the acuity of both eyes, the patient will start to complain of double vision. These patients will benefit from the MR test and prismatic control.

The MR consists of a series of strong, convex/plano-convex (plus) cylindrical red glass rods side by side, which convert the appearance of a white spot of light into a red streak. When the rods are orientated vertically, the streak will be

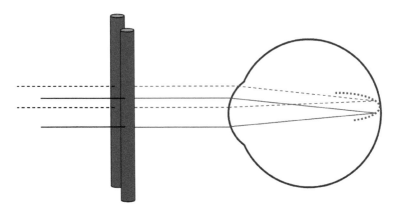

Figure 4.13 Optics of the Maddox rod. Vertical axis of the cylinders produces a horizontal line and vice versa

horizontal and vice versa. Light from a distant source passes through the red cyls with no deviation in the same meridian as the axis of the cyls (since they have no power in the direction of their axis). Since there are multiple red rods, this gives a single red line on the retina and is perceived (see Figure 4.13). Light rays in other meridians are converged by these powerful rods to a point focus just in front of the eye that is too close for it to be appreciated (this is not seen).

By placing the MR in front of one eye, whilst the patient fixates at a distant white light, the two eyes are dissociated, since one eye stares at the red line whilst the other stares at the white light. If orthophoric, the red line will appear to pass through the white light when the red line is orientated either vertically or horizontally. If there is a horizontal phoria, when the red line is orientated vertically (rods horizontal), the red line will appear to one side. If there is a vertical phoria when the red line is orientated horizontally (rods vertical), the red line will appear either above or below the white light.

This may sound complex, but with practice, the MR test can be completed in less than 1 minute with ease. Remember that corrective prisms have their apex directed in the direction of eye deviation.

The distant cover test is useful to do prior to the MR test, since it gives an objective starting point to which the MR test's subjective result should match. Note that the distant cover test should normally be followed by the near cover test (i.e. cover test with near target as fixation), but in the context of the MR, this is not really necessary, since you are trying to establish whether or not prisms are required for a distance prescription.

Now turn the room lights down. With the binocular, distance prescription in place, ask the patient to fixate at a distant white dot light (somebody holding a pen-torch at the end of the room is sufficient if no white dot light is in the light box).

Hold the MR in front of the right eye, with the bars orientated horizontally and ask the patient if they can see a vertical red line. If they cannot, occlude their left eye momentarily and the red line is normally seen. If persistently unable to see the red line with both eyes uncovered, the patient is likely to be suppressing that eye due to longstanding strabismus.

Ask them if the red line is to the right, left, or straight through the white dot. If the line goes through the white dot, then no prismatic correction in the horizontal plane is required (Figure 4.14a).

If the line is to the right, they have an esophoria (Figure 4.14b), and BO prisms should be placed in front of the left eye until the red line is through the white spot. In theory, a BO prism could also be placed in front of the right eye to correct an esophoria, but since the MR is in front of the right eye, it is easier to place prisms in front of the left.

If the line is to the left, they have an exophoria (Figure 4.14c), and BI prisms should be placed in front of the left eye until the red line is through the white spot. Again, this could also be corrected with a BI prism in front of the right eye, but since the MR is in front of the right eye, it is easier to place prisms in front of the left eye.

A 3 pd lens can be used first to try to shift the position of the red line to pass through the white spot or, if overcorrected, to pass over to the other side. In patients without diplopia, 3 pd is usually sufficient to shift the line and confirms that no prisms need to be incorporated into the spectacle prescription. In patients with diplopia, more than 3 pd will probably be required to shift the red line to pass through the white spot. The resultant prismatic correction should then be shared between the two eyes. For example, if 8 pd BO is required to correct an esodeviation, 4 pd BO in front of the right eye and 4 pd BO in front of the left eye should be prescribed. If 13 pd BI is required to correct an exodeviation, 7 pd BI in front of the right eye and 6 pd BI in front of the left eye should be prescribed.

Now hold the MR in front of the right eye with the rods orientated vertically and ask the patient if they can see a horizontal red line. Ask them if the red line is above, below, or straight through the white light.

If the line goes through the white dot, then no prismatic correction in the vertical plane is required (Figure 4.14d).

If the line lies above the white dot (Figure 4.14e), they have a left hyperphoria or alternatively a right hypophoria. This can be corrected with a BD prism in front of the left eye. This could also be corrected with a BU prism in front of the right eye.

If the line lies below the white dot (Figure 4.14f), they have a left hypophoria (or a right hyperphoria), which can be corrected with a BU prism in front of the left eye (or a BD prism in front of the right eye).

Again, for vertical deviations, a 3 prism dioptre lens can be used, but note that patients are generally more sensitive to vertical deviations. For example, a 3 prism dioptre deviation in the horizontal plane is usually fused and doesn't result in symptomatic diplopia, whereas 3 prism dioptres in the vertical plane may not be fused and the patient may have diplopia. If a vertical prismatic correction is required, then again this should be shared between the two eyes, but unlike horizontal deviations, for vertical deviations, the prisms are orientated in opposite directions. For example, a 5 prism dioptre left hyperdeviation can be managed

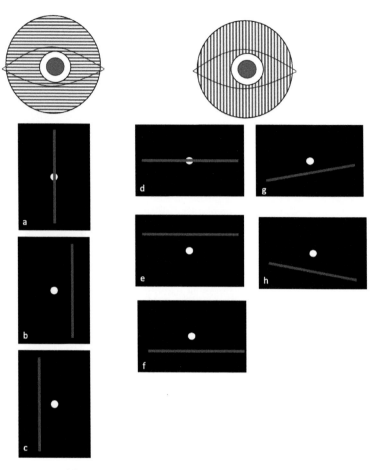

Figure 4.14 Possible outcomes of the Maddox rod over the right eye.
(a) Horizontal orthophoria, (b) esophoria, (c) exophoria, (d) vertical orthophoria,
(e) hypophoria, (f) hyperphoria, (g) hyperphoria with excyclotorsion,
(h) hyperphoria with incyclotorsion

with 3 prism dioptres BD in front of the left eye and 2 prism dioptres BU in front of the right eye.

Finally, if the patient reports the line appears tilted or slanted with the rods oriented vertically, there is a degree of torsional deviation. Asking the patient which end is higher than the other indicates the direction of torsion. An excyclororted eye will perceive the MR line to be incyclotorted, so the right end of the line will be higher than the left. When accompanied by a hyperphoria (Figure 4.14g), this indicates a superior oblique underaction (cranial nerve IV palsy). An incyclotorted eye will perceive the MR line to be excyclotorted, so the left end of the line will be higher than the right. Incyclotorsion combined with hyperphoria (Figure 4.14h) indicates a skew deviation, and cerebellar or brainstem pathology should be investigated. To quantify the degree of torsion, the 'double Maddox Rod test' is performed, by placing an MR of different colours in front of each eye in the trial frame, both aligned in the same orientation. The MR is then rotated until the patient reports the two lines are parallel, simply reading off the angles from the cyl axis on the trial frame.

You may have realised that if the MR is placed in front of the right eye and the corrective prisms are then placed in front of the left eye, then the apex of the prism is always in the same direction that the patient reports the red line to appear, relative to the white dot:

•	Line to the left:	place prism with apex to left
•	Line to the right:	place prism with apex to right
•	Line above:	place prism with apex upwards
•	Line below:	place prism with apex downwards

Therefore, it is simple to place the MR in front of the right eye and use corrective prisms in front of the left eye with the apex pointing to where the red line lies. The only situation in which this is not possible is when the right eye has relatively poor best-corrected acuity (due to amblyopia or ocular pathology). In this case, the MR should be held in front of the left eye.

Near vision

'Accommodation' refers to the process of the focal point of the eye shifting from a distant target to a near target.

Patients who are presbyopic are unable to read clearly whilst wearing their distant spectacle prescription due to an inability to accommodate.

Presbyopia manifests at an earlier age in hypermetropes (from age 35 years) than in emmetropes (from age 40 years) and may never manifest in myopes.

Near vision is also improved by pupillary constriction, which increases the depth of focus. Adequate macular function is also vital for satisfactory near vision. For these reasons, checking near vision with good illumination is most helpful.

Given that patients will converge with near targets, they may also require a prismatic correction different to their distant correction (see section 'Prism cover test').

To estimate an initial near add, obtain a brief relevant history:

• their age
• whether they have had previous cataract surgery with an intraocular lens implant (pseudophakia)
• their activities of daily living that involve near visual tasks – reading, needle work, model making, etc., since this will alter their near working distance

Age	Near add
40–50 years	+1.00 to +1.50
50–60 years	+1.50 to +2.50
>60 years	+2.50 to +3.00
Pseudophakic	+2.50 to +3.00

You may need to adjust the trial frame so that the trial lenses are centred on the pupillary near centration distance, to avoid inducing any prism with the patient converging for near.

To assess near vision, ask the patient to hold the reading chart at their comfortable near working distance for the near task they would like correction for

- reading – typically about 33cm
- needle work/model making, etc. – may be much closer and therefore require a greater near add
- computer work – such an intermediate distance may require a weaker add to the distant prescription, relative to full near correction required for reading

Occlude the left eye and ask them to read the smallest print they can on the N-Series reading chart held at their working distance. Now add the appropriate near plus lens and record the corrected near acuity (aiming for N5 or N6 in the absence of ocular disease).

Ask them to look at a letter, then ask:

Is the letter clearer 'with' [placing a +0.25 ds in front of their eye] *or without the lens* [remove the +0.25 ds], *or about the same?*

If they report that the letter is better with the lens, or about the same, then give the +0.25 ds and repeat until acuity is optimal.

Repeat the process for the left eye (occlude the right) and then check that the reading speed is good with both eyes not occluded.

The patient's near add is typically the same for both eyes, but this should still be checked as pre-presbyopes that have had unilateral cataract surgery will require a high near add in their pseudophakic eye and perhaps only a small near add in their phakic eye.

5

How to use a focimeter

FOCIMETER PRINCIPLES

The focimeter is used to measure the back vertex power of a lens. It is possible to establish the sphere, cyl (power and axis), and near add of a pair of bifocal spectacles. It can also be used to measure the amount and direction of prism that may have been incorporated into the lens. It is not so accurate at measuring the strength of varifocal spectacles.

The Refraction Certificate examination requires candidates to use the focimeter. In 5 minutes, you'll be expected to record the distance and near prescription for a pair of bifocal spectacles.

Focimeters consist of a collimating lens which makes diverging light rays from an illuminated target parallel, as well as a telescope that focuses the target onto a graticule (see Figure 5.1). The focused target can then be observed through a viewing system. The target will only be focused on the graticule once the light rays entering the telescope are parallel, so when a test lens is placed on the focimeter at the lens rest, the distance of the target from the collimating lens has to be altered until the light rays entering the telescope are parallel and the light rays of the target are focused onto the graticule. This gives a power value that is noted from a calibrated scale. There are different types of focimeter but they all work using this principle. Generally, two types are used in the Refraction Certificate, which are based on their illuminated targets – the ring of dots and the cross-line targets. It is important to get acquainted with both to avoid any unpleasant surprises on the day of the exam, as there will not be a choice! This chapter will cover both.

Before using the focimeter, look at the spectacles and note that if they are bifocal, then a near add value will also be required. Quickly note that if they minify an object, then they will be the spectacles of a myope (minus lens), whereas if they magnify an object, then they will be the spectacles of a hypermetrope (plus lens).

As one looks through the eyepiece, there are four features that should be noted. The protractor, see Figure 5.2a, and graticule, see Figure 5.2b, together determine the axis of the cylinder of the lens through rotating the graticule about 180 degrees, as well as the direction of the base of any incorporated. Each line of the graticule corresponds to 1 prism dioptre to measure the size of the incorporated prism. The target

DOI: 10.1201/9781003329329-5

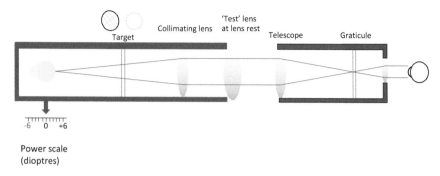

Figure 5.1 Optics of a focimeter

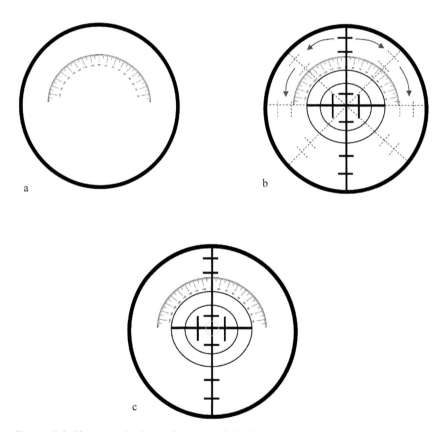

Figure 5.2 Showing the basic features of the focimeter through the eyepiece.
(a) The protractor, (b) the graticule, (c) the target

is shown as the ring of dots in Figure 5.2c. Finally, the dioptric power scale allows the power of the lens to be recorded.

RECORDING DISTANCE PRESCRIPTION

Turn the focimeter on and set the power wheel to zero. Then turn the viewing eyepiece fully anticlockwise, look down the eyepiece, and turn it clockwise until the dots and graticule are in focus (this reduces instrument accommodation which will give a false recording). It's also important to perform this procedure with both eyes open as using one eye only will also induce instrument accommodation whilst focusing.

Place the spectacles on the lens shelf with the arms facing backwards (see Figure 5.3) to ensure that the focimeter measures the back vertex power of the lens. Conventionally, the distance then near prescription is established for the right lens, and then repeated for the left lens.

If the glasses are bifocals, check that the upper distance segment is orientated on the focimeter. You may need to move the lens around until the target is centralised on the graticule. If this is not possible, it is due to a prism in the lens (see 'Recording the prismatic correction').

Ring of dots target

Once the spectacles are placed on the focimeter, a ring of dots is only seen if the lens only contains a sphere and when the collimating lens is focused (see Figure 5.2c). Therefore, rotate the focusing wheel until a crisp ring of dots is seen, and then note the power value and sign (+ or –) on the wheel. This will give the distance spherical prescription.

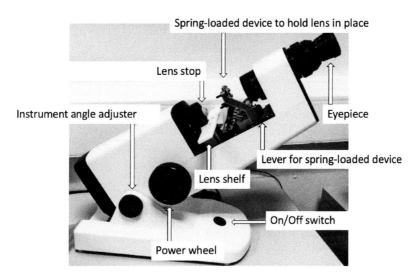

Figure 5.3 Focimeter labelled by component

As with most cases, the prescription will have an astigmatic element, so rather than a ring of dots, a ring of lines is observed. Turning the focusing wheel will bring these lines into focus, and turning the wheel further will bring a set of perpendicular lines into focus (the previous lines will become blurred or disappear). The length of the lines correlates with the amount of astigmatism, so the greater the difference in the powers between the two principal meridians, the longer the lines. It is necessary to adjust the axis of the graticule so that the lines are made fine and linear. Once the axis has been corrected, turn the focusing wheel to bring the lines into sharp focus. Failure to first match the axis will result in a spherical blur. Record the power and the axis – this is the value of the cylindrical component in one of the two principal meridians. Then, turn the focusing wheel until the perpendicular lines appear. Again, fine-tune the axis of the graticule until the lines are linear and then alter the power wheel until in sharp focus. Record the power and axis of this perpendicular principal meridian.

It is quite simple to convert the two cyl recordings into a spectacle prescription. If working in plus cyls:

- the sphere is the most negative recording
- the cyl is plus and is the **difference** between the two recordings
- the axis is the same as the most plus recording

Here's a worked example:

The first reading on the left in Figure 5.4a is the less positive sphere value of + 0.50 D at 025. Rotating the mires less than 90 degrees will result in a blurred target (see Figure 5.4b). Rotation of 90 degrees brings the next principal meridian into focus at +1.75D at 115 (see Figure 5.4c). The cyl is the difference between the two in plus form: +1.25 D, and the axis is taken from the second more plus value, in this case 115. The prescription therefore reads +0.5 / +1.25 x 115.

If working in minus cyl:

- The sphere is the most positive recording
- The cyl is negative and is the **difference** between the two recordings
- The axis is the same as the second (more negative) reading

TWO CYL RECORDINGS FROM FOCIMETER		PRESCRIPTION (NEGATIVE AND PLUS CYL FORMS)
3.00 x 030	–2.00 x 120	+3.00 /–5.00 x 120 –2.00 / +5.00 x 030
–1.75 x 145	–3.25 x 055	–1.75 / –1.50 x 055 –3.25 / +1.50 x 145
+1.50 x 060	+6.25 x 150	+6.25 / –4.75 x 060 +1.50 / +4.75 x 150

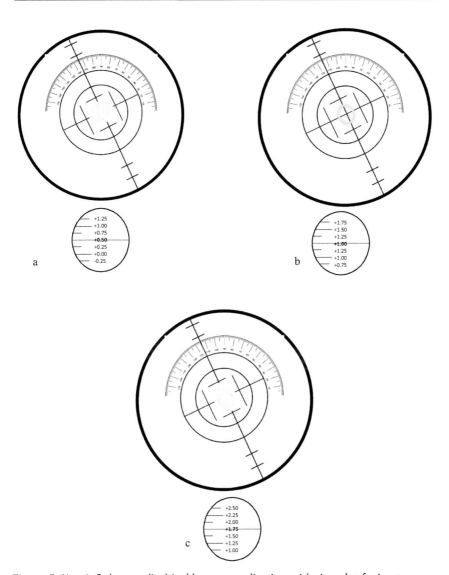

Figure 5.4(a–c) Sphero-cylindrical lens neutralisation with ring-dot focimeter

Here are some other examples:

Cross-line target

The cross-line target consists of two sets of three lines perpendicular to one another, one set thin and one thick. The same principles apply to the ring-dot target regarding the protractor, graticule, and power scale. Similarly, for spherical lenses, all lines will come into focus at the same time, see Figure 5.5.

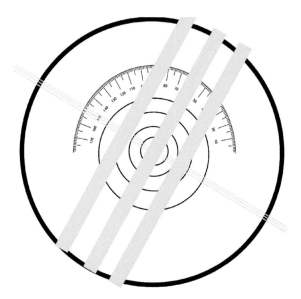

Figure 5.5 Spherical cross-line target

For sphero-cylindrical lenses, the two sets of lines will not focus at the same time. Again, we'll work in negative cyl but it's easy enough to convert to positive cyl, which we'll come onto. Turn the power wheel to a high positive value. Slowly reduce the power scale and adjust the axis by rotating the graticule until one set of lines comes into focus. This more positive principal meridian is the sphere value. Continue reducing until the perpendicular set of lines comes into focus. There is no need to rotate the graticule any further, and you can simply read off the axis of the second principal meridian.

If working in negative cyl:

- the sphere is the more positive dioptric power value
- the cyl is the **difference** between the two readings in negative form
- the axis is the value of the second (more negative) reading

Another worked example:

The first set of lines comes into focus at –1.75 D at 060 (see Figure 5.6a). This less positive meridian is our sphere value. The next set of lines comes into focus at +0.50 D at 150 (Figure 5.6b). The cyl value in plus form is the difference of the two: +2.25 dioptres. The axis is taken from the second, more plus meridian, 150. Our prescription therefore is –1.75 / +2.25 x 150.

If working in minus cyl:

- The sphere is the most positive recording
- The cyl is negative and is the **difference** between the two recordings
- The axis is the same as the second (more negative) reading

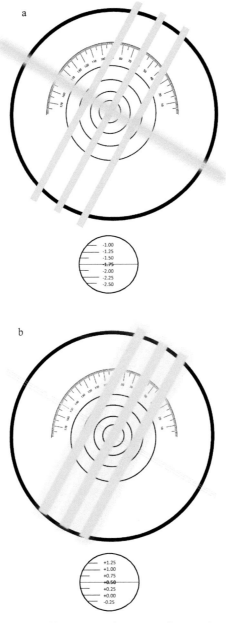

Figure 5.6 Sphero-cylindrical lens neutralisation with cross-line focimeter

Note that the focimeter records the cyl axis and not the orientation of the cyl power (perpendicular to axis). This is important to appreciate if using power crosses to obtain the prescription, rather than the simple three-step process described here.

For example, if the two cyl recordings from the focimeter are +3.00 x 135 and –1.75 x 045, this would give the following power cross:

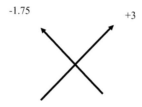

This gives –1.75 / +4.75 x 135 (equivalent to +3.00 / –4.75 x 045).

See Chapter 4, section 'Power Crosses', to see how to obtain the prescription from the power cross. Although academically, it is useful to appreciate power crosses, you may well find it simpler to use the three-step rule detailed above.

Most focimeters have a dioptric range of –25.00 to +25.00 dioptres. Should the test lens fall outside this, and the target cannot be brought into focus, then placing a spherical trial lens of opposite sign against the back vertex of the lens. For example, placing a +5.0 ds lens against the back vertex of a –25ds test lens, will be neutralised at –20.0 on the focimetry power scale.

Recording near add value

To measure the near add of the bifocal segment, move the spectacles so that the lower near segment is orientated on the focimeter. Rotate the power wheel until the dots (or lines in the case of astigmatism) are in focus and record the power. Subtract the distance prescription from this near value to give the near add.

For example, if the dots are in sharp focus at –3.00 ds for the distance segment and –1.50 ds for the near segment, then the near add will be +1.50 ds. When establishing the near add for a sphero-cylindrical lens (used to correct astigmatism), ensure that the lines brought into focus are at the same orientation as those lines used to give the power value for the distance that is subtracted from the near recording. For example, if the lines are in focus for the distance segment at +3.00 x 030 and –2.50 x 120, and the 030 line is in focus at +5.00 for the near segment, then the near add is +2.00 ds. The 120 lines would then be in focus at –0.50 for the near segment.

In most cases, the near add value will be the same for each eye. However, do not assume this, since they may be the spectacles of a young patient that has had unilateral cataract surgery and hence needs no near add on one side and a pseudophakic near add for the other.

For high near adds, purists will argue that the spectacles should be rotated, since it should really be the difference between the distance back vertex power and the near front vertex power that gives the near add. However, this is often not easily done since the spectacle arms can clash with the front parts of the focimeter, and practically for most near adds keeping the spectacles with their back surface against the lens rest is normally adequate.

Recording the prismatic correction

When trying to centre the dots on the graticule, it may become apparent that the dots cannot be centralised. This is due to a prism being incorporated into the lens.

The dots will be deviated towards the base of the prism, since although prisms deviate images towards their apex, the focimeter eyepiece viewing system inverts this view. The power of the prism is equal to the number of spaces (denoted by the graticule) that the dots are deviated.

For example, if the dots are deviated by two spaces upwards, there is a 2 pd BU prism in that lens (see Figure 5.7a). If the dots are deviated by four spaces to the right when the right lens is being assessed, there is incorporated 4 pd BI prism (see Figure 5.7b).

Typically the prismatic correction is halved between the two lenses, and the bases will be in the same direction for horizontal deviations and opposite directions

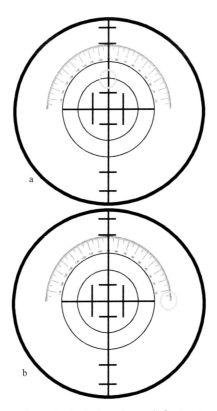

Figure 5.7 Measuring prismatic deviation through focimetry. (a) Lens with 2 pd base-up prism, (b) right lens with 4 pd base-in prism

for vertical deviations. For example, a 13 pd esodeviation will be corrected by a 6 pd BI correction in front of the right eye and 7 pd correction in front of the left eye. A 4 pd right hyperdeviation will be corrected by a 2 pd BD correction in front of the right eye and a 2 pd BU correction in front of the left eye. The apex of the correcting prism is always in the direction of deviation.

Symptomatic ocular deviations can be corrected by incorporating prisms into the spectacle prescription, which can be measured by the focimeter as described above. However, it is important to note that ocular deviations can also be controlled in another way – 'lens decentration'. This is where the optical axis of the lens is purposefully decentred relative to the patient's pupil. The prismatic power (prism dioptres) is equal to the power of the lens (dioptres) multiplied by the distance of decentration (cm). If this has been done, then it will still be possible to centre the image on the focimeter. Such prismatic correction could therefore be overlooked. The only way to detect lens decentration is by checking the lens for a marking that indicates this or by using a lens marker to mark the position of the pupil centre whilst the patient is wearing the spectacles. This mark should then be placed in the centre of the focimeter stop and any decentration will be evident. Fortunately, in the Refraction Certificate examination, since you are provided only with a pair of bifocal spectacles but not their owner, it is not expected to mark the pupil centre and assess for lens decentration.

6

Lens neutralisation

It is possible to establish the spectacle distance and near prescription (and also prismatic component) of a pair of bi-focal spectacles using a lens box by the principle of lens neutralisation. This estimate may not be as accurate as a focimeter; however, it is still a useful skill to have and one that is assessed in the Refraction Certificate examination.

Lens neutralisation uses lenses of equal but opposite power to neutralise a test spectacle lens so that there is no overall effect, as the combined net power will be zero. For example, a +2.50 ds spectacle is neutralised with a –2.50 ds lens. A 2 pd BO prism will be neutralised by a 2 pd BI prism.

First, to establish if the lens is minus or plus, complete the 'transverse test'. Draw a target or cross formed by two perpendicular lines. Pass the lens horizontally from left to right over the crossing lines. If the image of the lines moves in the same direction (left to right) as the sweep (*with*), then the lens is minus (see Figure 6.1a). If the image of the line moves in the opposite direction to the sweep (*against*), then the lens is plus (see Figure 6.1b).

With movement = *Minus* lens
Against movement = *Plus* lens

If the transverse test implies the test lens is minus, then place a plus lens (say + 3.00 ds) in direct contact and see if this eliminates the movement of the vertical line image. If the movement is still *with* the sweep, then try a more plus lens; if it is *against*, then try a less plus lens. The reverse is true for plus test lenses. Neutralisation occurs when the image of the crossed lines remains still as the lenses are swept across them horizontally.

Note that it is vital that lenses are held in close contact, since if they are held apart, then their effective power is altered. The trial lens should be held against the *back surface* of the test lens being investigated, since it is the back vertex power that we are measuring. If this is not possible, then it is reasonable to hold the trial lens against the front surface of the test lens. In this instance, with minus lenses for myopia, there is negligible difference between the back and front vertex powers, so little margin of error is introduced. Plus lenses have a weaker front vertex power than back vertex

DOI: 10.1201/9781003329329-6

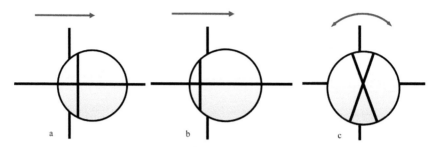

Figure 6.1 Transverse test and rotatory test. **(a)** *With* movement seen with minus lens, **(b)** *against* movement with plus lens, **(c)** scissoring seen with astigmatic lens

power, so this method will underestimate the power of the test lens, by –0.25 D for +5.00 lenses, and –0.75D for +10.00 +10 D lenses.

If there are different movements along the two principal meridians, this indicates a sphero-cylindrical test lens. This can be confirmed by rotating the lens clockwise and anti-clockwise. A spherical lens will not change the orientation of the lines, while a sphero-cylindrical lens will cause a scissoring of the lines as the lens is rotated clockwise and anti-clockwise (see Figure 6.1c). The principal meridians of the test lens should be identified and marked by rotating the lens until the crossed lines are perpendicular and continuous. Each principal meridian can then be neutralised as above.

Once the lens has been neutralised, the prismatic component (if present) can be neutralised in the same fashion by the application of equal and opposite prisms. Images viewed through a prism are displaced towards their apex. Hence a 3 pd BU prism will shift the image downwards and be neutralised by a 3 pd BD prism. Neutralisation occurs when the image is not shifted at all by the combined prisms.

7

Final tips for the exam

MORE THAN TWO MONTHS BEFORE THE EXAM

Read this book!

Read the Refraction Examination Certificate Application details very carefully and email the Royal College if you have any uncertainty about what is expected of you.

Consider attending a course on refraction. This will no doubt be helpful, but they are often expensive and are absolutely no substitute for refracting yourself.

Organise study leave not just for the exam, but for the week before the exam during which time you must refract intensively.

Get refracting! The retinoscopy simulators offer an excellent starting point and compose 40% of the exam stations. Familiarise yourself with the iPad answer submission format (see Appendix 1). You'll find it can take between 60 and 90 seconds to input your answers for every 5-minute station, so try and keep this to a minimum and be sure to set sufficient time aside.

Get well acquainted with the optometrists in your department. Not only are they often the friendliest folk in the hospital but they also are an excellent source of advice, critiquing and fine-tuning your retinoscopy technique.

Get your own retinoscope or borrow one so that its use becomes second nature. Borrow a decent trial frame and Jackson Cross Cylinder.

ONE MONTH BEFORE THE EXAM

You'll probably by now have realised that the main limitation to practising is obtaining a free room and a subject to refract. It does not take long to refract everybody in the department, so you'll need to look elsewhere.

Try all staff, so this includes medical, nursing, health care assistants, students, and administrative staff. Then try family members of staff – husbands and wives are often keen to have a free spectacle check! Therefore, whoever you refract, offer your service to their friends and family. You must however point out that you are not offering a full eye check and are not yet certified to prescribe spectacles – but you should be able to offer a reliable and free spectacle check. Often just chatting about the glasses somebody wears is useful for them. We found many satisfied customers! You may need to advertise by printing sheets and handing them around. Another trick is to refract the patients whilst they are waiting to be seen during the clinic.

Finally, consider booking people in advance into 30-minute slots to refract during your study week to ensure a final burst of resources!

ONE WEEK BEFORE THE EXAM

Really concentrate on getting your numbers up by refracting the people that you have booked into your free study week. Treat each refraction as a mock examination – time yourself!

It's really helpful to simulate a mock-style examination with the retinoscopy simulator. Ask a helpful colleague such as an optometrist in your department to spend an hour with you altering the power of the retinoscopy simulator and cyl lens inserted into the lens bracket, or spectacle lenses for lens neutralisation or focimetry. Practice inputting your answers into the iPad submission forms online.

Re-confirm that you understand the examination format.

Check you have all the things you will need to take with you which include:

- Your own retinoscope
- Place fresh batteries in your retinoscope and take a spare pair too
- Borrowed trial frame and Jackson Cross Cylinder
- Occluder, rule, and pen-torch (cover test)
- Passport or driving licence (required by examiners to check your identity)
- All the exam, accommodation, and travel details
- This book!

ON THE DAY

Get to the examination venue with plenty of time, having eaten and hydrated beforehand.

Prepare for starting with any station first.

Be consistent when recording your results – always use only positive cyls or only negative cyls (do not use both positive and negative cyl nomenclature).

All dioptric powers should be to two decimal places and have a clear + or – sign (e.g. +0.25, –1.50). The degrees sign (°) should be avoided and all axes should be to three significant figures (e.g. 045, 010, 135).

Keep your lenses tidy – it will annoy the examiners if they have to tidy up after you!

If you find yourself struggling with a retinoscopy reflex, don't just sit there persisting since prolonged retinoscopy sweeping is uncomfortable for the patient, induces accommodation, wastes limited time, and demonstrates your uncertainty to the examiners. No retinoscopy sweep burst should be more than a few seconds, so try to make a decision, and if unsure, simply come away and try a different lens.

Before formally starting, check that you are comfortable with the room set up (lighting, record sheet, check the equipment such as ensuring the focimeter is switched on and acuity chart if electronic, etc.) and ask questions if uncertain before that bell actually goes.

Finally, if a station has not gone to plan, cast it out of your mind and don't let it ruin your chances of success in the ones that follow, there is still everything to play for!

Good Luck!

8

Appendix

APPENDIX 1 – IPAD ANSWER SUBMISSION FORMS

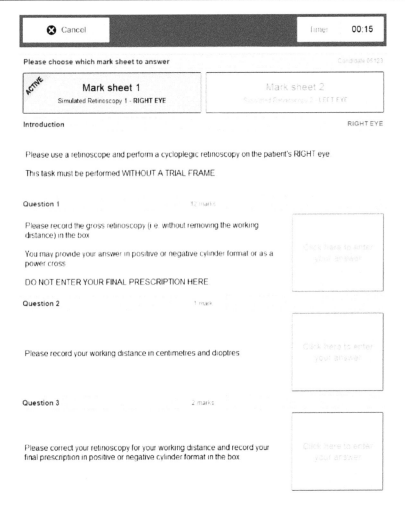

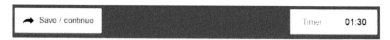

Save / continue   Timer   01:30

Question 1

Please record the gross retinoscopy (i.e. without removing the working distance) in the box.

You may provide your answer in positive or negative cylinder format or as a power cross

DO NOT ENTER YOUR FINAL PRESCRIPTION HERE

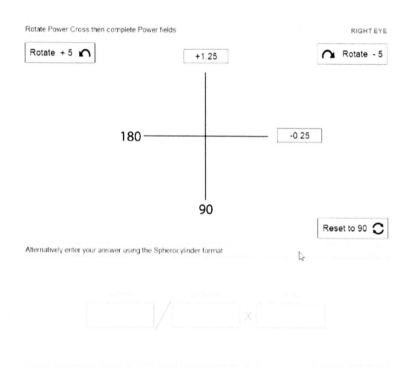

Rotate Power Cross then complete Power fields   RIGHT EYE

Rotate + 5   +1.25   Rotate - 5

180   -0.25

90

Reset to 90

Alternatively enter your answer using the Spherocylinder format

/   X

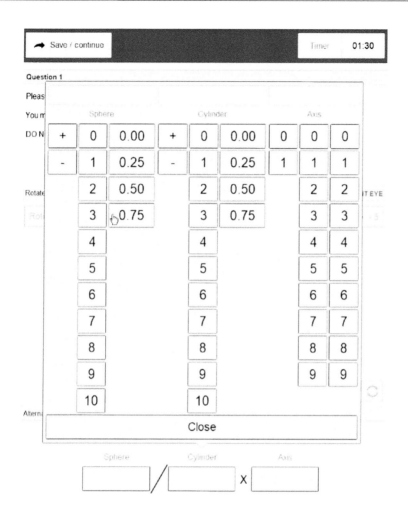

| Save / continue | | | | | | | Timer | 01:30 |

Question 1

Pleas

You m

DO N

Rotate

Altern

	Sphere			Cylinder			Axis	
+	0	0.00	+	0	0.00	0	0	0
-	1	0.25	-	1	0.25	1	1	1
	2	0.50		2	0.50		2	2
	3	0.75		3	0.75		3	3
	4			4			4	4
	5			5			5	5
	6			6			6	6
	7			7			7	7
	8			8			8	8
	9			9			9	9
	10			10				

Close

Sphere   Cylinder   Axis

/   X

APPENDIX 2 – THE RETINOSCOPE

There are two types of retinoscopes – slit and spot. Slit retinoscopes are far more common in ophthalmic outpatient departments, so the principles of the slit retinoscope are detailed here.

A retinoscope consists of a light source and a mirror with a viewing hole in it so the observer when looking through the hole can observe whatever is illuminated.

When the handle of the slit retinoscope is fully down, a linear light is produced (the scope slit). With the cuff down (correct position; Figure A2.1), a condensing lens between the light and mirror allows diverging rays to exit the retinoscope. With the cuff upwards, the condensing lens is moved to a different position to give converging rays.

As the scope slit is swept across the pupil, light entering the patient's eye is reflected by the retina and is then refracted by their eye before being observed by the practitioner through the viewing hole of the retinoscope. The quality of the light reflex depends upon the following factors:

- cuff position
- working distance
- refractive state of patient's eye
- scope slit orientation and direction of sweep

By ensuring that the cuff is fully down, the working distance is known and the scope slit orientation and direction of sweep controlled, it is possible for the practitioner to obtain an objective refraction for the patient's eye by interspersing various trial lenses in order to neutralise the retinoscopy reflex (see Chapter 4).

The optics of the retinoscope can be detailed further by considering how the retina is illuminated ('illumination stage'), how an image of the illuminated retina is formed at the patient's far point ('reflex stage'), and how the image at the far-point is located by moving the illumination across the retina and noting the reflex quality ('projection stage').

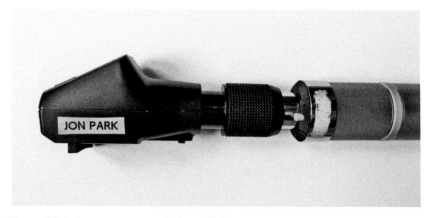

Figure A2.1 A retinoscope with the cuff down

This is beyond the scope of this refraction handbook, and we recommend that for further detailed optics information, you refer to this excellent book, which is also very useful for the Part I Fellowship Examination: Elkington AR, Frank HJ, Greaney MJ. *Clinical Optics*. Blackwell Publishing.

Index

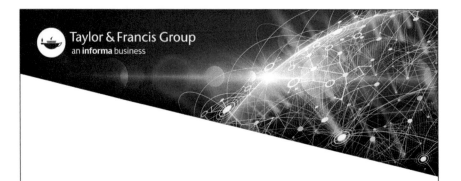